# Outsourcing the Womb

## France Winddance Twine

A quiet revolution has been taking place during the past three decades. The way children enter families has changed radically among upper middle class families. In the 1980s infertility increasingly became defined as a medical problem that could be solved with assisted reproductive technologies (ART) such as in vitro fertilization and embryo transfers rather than through adoption. As well, third parties, referred to as surrogates, are hired to assist individuals and/or couples who wish to conceive a child with whom they share a genetic tie. This has resulted in a "surrogate baby boom." This book provides a critical introduction to the global surrogacy market. A comparative analysis of the assisted reproductive technology and surrogacy industry in Egypt, Israel, India, and the United States disentangles the intersecting roles of race, religion, class inequality, religious law, and global capitalism and raises policy questions.

**France Winddance Twine** is a Professor of Sociology at the University of California in Santa Barbara. She is a consulting editor for *Ethnic and Racial Studies*. She teaches courses on race/class/gender, critical race theory, and qualitative research methods.

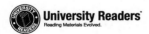
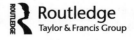

**University Readers**
Reading Materials Evolved.

THE SOCIAL ISSUES
COLLECTION™

**Routledge**
Taylor & Francis Group

# Framing 21st Century Social Issues

The goal of this new, unique Series is to offer readable, teachable "thinking frames" on today's social problems and social issues by leading scholars. These are available for view on http://routledge.custom gateway.com/routledge-social-issues.html.

For instructors teaching a wide range of courses in the social sciences, the Routledge *Social Issues Collection* now offers the best of both worlds: originally written short texts that provide "overviews" to important social issues *as well as* teachable excerpts from larger works previously published by Routledge and other presses.

As an instructor, click to the website to view the library and decide how to build your custom anthology and which thinking frames to assign. Students can choose to receive the assigned materials in print and/or electronic formats at an affordable price.

**Body Problems**
Running and Living Long in a Fast-Food Society
*Ben Agger*

**Sex, Drugs, and Death**
Addressing Youth Problems in American Society
*Tammy Anderson*

**The Stupidity Epidemic**
Worrying About Students, Schools, and America's Future
*Joel Best*

**Empire Versus Democracy**
The Triumph of Corporate and Military Power
*Carl Boggs*

**Contentious Identities**
Ethnic, Religious, and Nationalist Conflicts in Today's World
*Daniel Chirot*

**The Future of Higher Education**
*Dan Clawson and Max Page*

**Waste and Consumption**
Capitalism, the Environment, and the Life of Things
*Simonetta Falasca-Zamponi*

**Rapid Climate Change**
Causes, Consequences, and Solutions
*Scott G. McNall*

**The Problem of Emotions in Societies**
*Jonathan H. Turner*

**Outsourcing the Womb**
Race, Class, and Gestational Surrogacy in a Global Market
*France Winddance Twine*

**Changing Times for Black Professionals**
*Adia Harvey Wingfield*

**Why Nations Go to War**
A Sociology of Military Conflict
*Mark Worrell*

# Outsourcing the Womb
## Race, Class, and Gestational Surrogacy in a Global Market

# France Winddance Twine
University of California, Santa Barbara

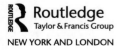
Routledge
Taylor & Francis Group

NEW YORK AND LONDON

First published 2011
by Routledge
270 Madison Avenue, New York, NY 10016

Simultaneously published in the UK
by Routledge
2 Park Square, Milton Park, Abingdon, Oxon OX14 4RN

*Routledge is an imprint of the Taylor & Francis Group, an informa business*

Typeset in Garamond and Gill Sans by EvS Communication Networx, Inc.

*Library of Congress Cataloging in Publication Data*
Twine, France Winddance, 1960-
Outsourcing the womb : race, class, and gestational surrogacy in a global market / France Winddance Twine.
p. cm. — (Framing 21st century social issues)
Includes bibliographical references and index.
1. Surrogate motherhood. 2. Surrogate motherhood—Economic aspects.
3. Human reproductive technology—Social aspects. I. Title.
HQ759.5.T95 2011
306.874'3—dc22
2010052906

ISBN13: 978-0-415-89202-5 (pbk)
ISBN13: 978-0-203-83420-6 (ebk)

# Contents

# Series Foreword

The world in the early 21st century is beset with problems—a troubled economy, global warming, oil spills, religious and national conflict, poverty, HIV, health problems associated with sedentary lifestyles. Virtually no nation is exempt, and everyone, even in affluent countries, feels the impact of these global issues.

Since its inception in the 19th century, sociology has been the academic discipline dedicated to analyzing social problems. It is still so today. Sociologists offer not only diagnoses; they glimpse solutions, which they then offer to policy makers and citizens who work for a better world. Sociology played a major role in the civil rights movement during the 1960s in helping us to understand racial inequalities and prejudice, and it can play a major role today as we grapple with old and new issues.

This series builds on the giants of sociology, such as Weber, Durkheim, Marx, Parsons, Mills. It uses their frames, and newer ones, to focus on particular issues of contemporary concern. These books are about the nuts and bolts of social problems, but they are equally about the frames through which we analyze these problems. It is clear by now that there is no single correct way to view the world, but only paradigms, models, which function as lenses through which we peer. For example, in analyzing oil spills and environmental pollution, we can use a frame that views such outcomes as unfortunate results of a reasonable effort to harvest fossil fuels. "Drill, baby, drill" sometimes involves certain costs as pipelines rupture and oil spews forth. Or we could analyze these environmental crises as inevitable outcomes of our effort to dominate nature in the interest of profit. The first frame would solve oil spills with better environmental protection measures and clean-ups, while the second frame would attempt to prevent them altogether, perhaps shifting away from the use of petroleum and natural gas and toward alternative energies that are "green."

These books introduce various frames such as these for viewing social problems. They also highlight debates between social scientists who frame problems differently. The books suggest solutions, both on the macro and micro levels. That is, they suggest what new policies might entail, and they also identify ways in which people, from the ground level, can work toward a better world, changing themselves and their lives and families and providing models of change for others.

Readers do not need an extensive background in academic sociology to benefit from these books. Each book is student-friendly in that we provide glossaries of terms for the uninitiated that are keyed to bolded terms in the text. Each chapter ends with questions for further thought and discussion. The level of each book is accessible to undergraduate students, even as these books offer sophisticated and innovative analyses.

Twine has written a pioneering book on "reproductive tourism"—where infertile couples use birthing surrogates in the United States and India. She analyzes this rapidly growing market in terms of the exploitation of usually poor women in these two countries who, in effect, rent their wombs in order to service the fertility needs of more affluent couples. She notes that there are virtually no protections afforded these surrogates and she documents aspects of economic exploitation involved in this unusual approach to forming families. This book is a contribution to scholarship on fertility, families, and globalization.

# Preface

A quiet revolution has been taking place during the past three decades. The way that children enter families has changed radically, especially among upper middle class families who have fertility problems in the United States. Asexual or "assisted conception" involving medical technologies such as in vitro fertilization and embryo transfers has replaced sexual reproduction (and adoption) for infertile heterosexual couples and for same sex couples who need assistance in forming families. Wealthier families are increasingly selecting surrogacy instead of adoption as a method for acquiring children with whom they have a genetic tie. In 1987 Genea Corea wrote, "The rise of the surrogate industry does not take place in isolation. It is part of the industrialization of reproduction. It is part of the opening up of the 'reproductive supermarket'."

This book provides a critical examination of assisted reproductive technologies (ART) and the gestational surrogacy industry in a global market. Gestational surrogacy involves ART with the use of third parties, referred to as surrogates, to assist individuals and/or couples who wish to conceive a child with whom they have a genetic tie. This has resulted in a "surrogate baby boom." In the 1980s infertility increasingly became defined as a medical problem that could be solved with ART rather than through adoption. These assisted reproductive technologies have challenged the idea of "natural" reproduction and of the meaning of parenthood.

Although infertility is a global health issue that affects millions of people worldwide there is ambivalence and anxiety about the commercial use of assisted reproductive technologies and particularly gestational surrogacy. While most industrialized nations ban commercial surrogacy others such as Brazil, Israel, and the United Kingdom have established regulatory regimes or partial bans to control access to it. The surrogacy market is unregulated by the United States government, leaving it up to individual states to develop regulatory policies. The legal restrictions placed on surrogacy in most of Europe and Asia have enabled California to be the global destination of choice for reproductive tourists.

The global market for fertility therapies is structured by racial, class, and economic inequalities. The World Health Organization (WHO) estimates, that, on average, at least one in every ten couples in developing countries experiences some form of infertility during their reproductive lives. Yet access to reproductive health and assisted reproductive services remains restricted to a small percentage of people who have the resources to purchase these technologies. This book provides a comparative analysis of the use of assisted reproductive technologies in Egypt, India, Israel, and the United States. By providing a comparative analysis of this industry across several national contexts the book disentangles the roles that race, religion, class inequality, religious law, and global capitalism play in the surrogacy market. This book draws on case studies from Egypt, India, Israel, and the United States to examine the ways that surrogacy is managed by women employed in this industry and to illuminate the ways that race, class, gender, religion, nationality, and legal regimes structure the experiences of contract pregnancy. A comparative analysis of this industry in both developing nations such as India as well as the United States and Israel provides a more compelling, critical and complex view of a form of women's labor that is being outsourced and constitutes a growing segment of the medical tourism industry.

This book has three goals: 1) provide an intersectional analysis of the ways that racism, class inequalities, colonial legacies, religious beliefs, and transnational capitalism structure the use of assisted reproductive technologies and gestational surrogacy; 2) analyse the ethical, legal, and public policy debates around reproductive labor, and 3) provide a comparative analysis of the experiences of gestational surrogates who are employed in this global market. This book provides an intersectional frame of analysis in which multiple forms of social inequality and power differences become institutionalized in this market and restrict the access of some individuals and families while privileging others. This book concludes with a discussion of "reproductive justice." What would reproductive justice look like in this global market?

# Acknowledgments

A book is never the product of one person, but is always a collaboration. A number of people contributed in large and small ways to the completion of this book. First and foremost I thank Ben Agger for encouraging me to write it. Elizabeth Baur worked enthusiastically and tirelessly as a research assistant for me and without her support I would not have completed this in a timely manner. I received numerous forms of support from Linda Jack, Susan Pilch, Tricia Sota, Ravi Shivanna, Iris Wilson, and Susan Mattos at the Center for Advanced Study in Behavioral Sciences when I embarked on the study of the surrogacy industry.

I have been fortunate to have the emotional support, friendship, and love of Debbie Rogow, Howard Winant, Paul Amar, Lisa Hajjar, and Constance Penley. Tanya Golash-Boza, Anita Davis-Twine, Kristin Thornton-Twine, Joseph Jewell, Seena Brodnax-Anderson, Jacquelyn Nassy Brown, Melissa MacDonald, and Sally Russ all provided cheerleading when I needed that extra push. Finally I thank Allan Cronin, Candace Assassi, Angela Picerni, and Evely Laser Shlensky who made it possible for me to complete this book.

# 1:  The Industrial Womb

On January 3, 2008, Judith Warner published "Outsourced Wombs" in a blog in *The New York Times*. Warner raises ethical questions about the complexities of transnational gestational surrogacy, a growing segment of the **reproductive tourism** industry. Increasingly women and couples from the United States and Europe have begun traveling to India to hire women at discount rates to gestate and deliver babies for a fraction of what it would cost in the United States. They are, like companies that outsource labor to other countries, traveling to purchase a cheaper source of reproductive labor. In this blog Warner made references to the dystopic fiction of Aldous Huxley's *Brave New World* and Margaret Atwood's *A Handmaid's Tale* in which reproduction is imagined as an industrial or outsourced procedure.

The print version of the *American Heritage Dictionary* defines **outsourcing** as "To farm out (work) for example to an outside provider or manufacturer to cut costs" (1996: 1287). In recent years, the term outsourcing has been increasingly used by feminists and others to refer to the reproductive labor performed by pregnant women who are providing a form of contract labor—renting their wombs out to women whom they may not even meet to gestate babies to whom they have no genetic tie. **Gestational surrogacy** is a form of industrial labor that has not been previously considered by economists or economic sociologists in their discussions of outsourcing yet it represents a growing segment of the reproductive tourism or medical tourism market.

Women, typically the mothers of young children and from poor or lower middle class backgrounds, are selling their reproductive labor on an increasingly competitive global market. The comments of the hundreds of people who responded to Warner's blog reflect the mixture of ambivalence, anxiety, genetic entitlement, and a range of competing ethical attitudes towards this form of **commercial pregnancy** in the fertility industry.

On April 8, 2008, the cover story for *Newsweek* magazine featured the pregnant belly of an anonymous White woman. The cover read, "Womb for Rent: The Complex World of Surrogate Mothers." We learn that military wives are targeted by agencies as potential **surrogates**: "Surrogate agencies target the population by dropping leaflets in the mailboxes of military housing complexes such as those around San Diego's Camp Pendleton and placing ads in on-base publications such as *Military Times* and *Military*

*Spouse*" (Ali and Kelley 2008: 48). The *Newsweek* article addressed an issue that is central to sociologists interested in new family formations and social inequality.[1]

"Are there any ethical limits on what one person may pay another to do? It is a question that rarely arises in the world of normal commerce, even in the modern service economy," wrote Roger Rosenblatt in 1987. Rosenblatt raised questions that remain the subject of controversy in academic, legal, public policy, and ethical debates about surrogacy and **assisted reproductive technologies** (ART). Although profound ambivalence and anxieties continue to surround the practice of commercial surrogacy in the United States, a laissez-faire capitalist consumer culture has enabled surrogacy to become a major industry attracting a global clientele. What is surprising is not that surrogacy has generated controversy, but that it has generated less controversy than abortion, contraception and same sex marriage—all issues used by politicians during every campaign season to generate support, raise financing and to negotiate their image. Surrogacy has yet to become a high-profile campaign issue. How can we understand the ethical debates around surrogacy?

What role should the state play in providing individuals and families with access to reproductive technologies? What criteria should be used to determine who "deserves" to have assisted conception? What role, if any, should private for-profit agencies play in assisted conception? Do unmarried women have a right to **in vitro fertilization** (IVF), assisted reproductive technology and to purchase sperm? What restrictions should be placed on ART? What role should religious beliefs play in access to and utilization of these assistive reproductive technologies? Should the U.S. pass federal legislation to protect the bodily integrity and rights of commercial surrogates?

Why does commercial surrogacy generate anxieties, ambivalence, controversy and hostility, yet remain legal in many countries? Why is surrogacy banned in most countries? A critical analysis of gestational surrogacy requires an analysis of the ways that the moral, social, political, legal, and religious contexts shape its interpretation and implementation.

This book provides an introduction to the global industry of commercial surrogacy. The gestational surrogacy industry, a growing segment of the global medical tourism industry, assists individuals and families in conceiving and acquiring children to form families. This transnational profit-driven industry has generated controversy, legislation, and a number of ethical questions that are troubling for sociologists of race,

---

1 According to this article, "Military wives who do decide to become surrogates can earn more with one pregnancy than their husbands' annual base pay (with ranges for new enlistees from $16,080 to $28,900)" (Ali and Kelley 2008: 48). Military wives are also "attractive candidates because of their health insurance, Tricare, which is provided by three different companies—Humana, Tri-West and Health Net Federal Services. And it has some of the most comprehensive coverage for surrogates in the industry" (2008: 48).

gender, and class inequality. Who should have access to these technologies? Should the state provide funding for ART to families who lack the resources to pay for them? How are racial, class, social, and other inequalities reinforced, reinscribed, and reproduced via these technologies? How do religious beliefs inform the transfer and utilization of these technologies? How do these technologies reinforce racial and ethnic boundaries? How is the problem of infertility conceptualized? Is it a personal problem? A public health problem? What are the competing frames? How do these interpretative frames reflect power inequities?

This book offers an original and critical examination of the use of ART and the commercial practice of gestational surrogacy. The ethical, moral, legal, religious, and policy debates surrounding the practice of gestational surrogacy are analyzed using the concept of **stratified reproduction**. Shellee Colen introduced the concept of stratified reproduction in her analysis of the relationships between West Indian migrant women working as childcare workers for U.S.-born White employers in New York. Colen defines stratified reproduction thus:

> By stratified reproduction, I mean that physical and social reproductive tasks are accomplished differently according to inequalities that are based on hierarchies of class, race, ethnicity, gender, place in a global economy ... The reproductive labor of bearing, raising, and socializing children ... is differentially experienced, valued and rewarded according to inequalities of access to material and social resources in particular historical and cultural contexts.
>
> (quoted in Ginsburg and Rapp 1995: 78)

Building upon the research of Shellee Colen, who conducted research among Black Caribbean domestic servants working on the upper West Side of Manhattan for New York White elites, I argue that gestational surrogacy is embedded in a transnational capitalist market that is structured by racial, ethnic, and class inequalities and by competing nation-state regulatory regimes. Consequently the same women who sell their reproductive labor and become reproductive service workers carrying pregnancies to term under labor contracts may not be able to afford basic health care for themselves or their own children once their labor contract expires. There is unequal access to assisted reproductive technologies in most countries because the cost is prohibitive and if it is not state funded then only elites and the upper middle classes can afford to purchase these services.

Do women have the right to rent out their wombs on a short-term basis? This is an area of controversy. Most industrialized countries either ban commercial surrogacy or highly regulate it. The United States is an exception. Poor women, underemployed women or women who want to supplement their income may rent their wombs out for a fee. However, the state plays a crucial role in the way the **gestational surrogates** and the intended parents experience this process. I will present case studies from Egypt,

Israel, and the United States to illuminate the way that race, class, religion, region, nationality, and legal regimes structure the commercial surrogacy industry.

There is a sparse but growing body of empirical literature on gestational surrogacy. Although vigorous debates have surrounded surrogacy, and the Baby M trial of the late 1980s generated media frenzy and resulted in a series of public debates that led to legislation restricting commercial surrogacy on the East coast, there are very few sociological studies of gestational surrogacy. The vast majority and most rigorous research has been done by anthropologists. There is a regional imbalance in that we have extensive participant observation and ethnographic research in the Middle East including Israel (Kahn 2000; Teman 2010) and Egypt (Inhorn 1995, 2003) and much less in the United States and Europe. A related body of literature has been focused upon the egg and sperm donation market, which is central to the assisted reproductive technology market (Ameling 2008).

This book examines the significant role of the state, capitalism, religion and nationality in the way that surrogacy is incorporated and utilized across national contexts in the United States, India, Israel, and Egypt. Drawing upon recent ethnographic studies, legal analyses, and philosophical debates this book examines the way that surrogacy reflects larger social problems around what constitutes parenthood and the meaning of "genetic" ties in an age of industrial pregnancy. We will move between national contexts to examine how ART and surrogacy are interpreted and the various responses to reproductive technologies.

## The Shift from Adoption to Assisted Reproduction

The decriminalization of abortion at the federal level dramatically altered the adoption market in the United States. After the 1973 Supreme Court case *Roe v. Wade* which legalized abortion and redefined it as a constitutional right to "privacy," the number of unmarried White women who gave birth to children declined. Abortion became more accessible, safer, and less stigmatized. The demand for White babies increased while the supply decreased. In other words, the supply chain was affected not only by abortion but also by the increasing refusal of White women to relinquish their children for adoption. A decade later, innovations in biomedicine increased the chances that people with resources could use in vitro fertilization to reproduce a child that had a genetic link. This altered expectations because now infertile couples who could afford it could seek IVF rather than adoption.

## From Test-Tube Babies to Gestational Surrogates

Aldous Huxley introduced the term "test-tube" babies in his 1932 novel *Brave New World*, in which he described a world where children were fertilized and incubated in artificial wombs. The term "test-tube" baby refers to fertilization that takes place outside of the womb. In vitro which literally means "in glass" refers to a biological process that ordinarily takes place within the body but occurs in a Petri dish or a glass laboratory receptacle.

On July 25, 1978, Louise Brown, the first "test-tube" baby was born in Oldham, England. Her parents were from working class backgrounds and had struggled to form a family for years. Three decades have passed since the first "test-tube" baby was born. At that time, this was still the stuff of science fiction novels and only barely believable. Today, according to the Center for Disease Control (2006), 1 percent of U.S. live births involved some assisted reproductive technologies. Embryos can be produced by in vitro fertilization using sperm and/or eggs from third parties (sellers or donors) and then transferred to a woman who is the gestational surrogate but may not be the intended parent. IVF has made it possible for same sex lesbian and gay male couples to have children biologically related to them. An embryo contains the full and unique genome of a potential human being, with all of his or her traits. Embryos are often frozen and stored for later use because the retrieval of eggs is an invasive and risky procedure. Consequently, doctors prefer to use hormones to overstimulate the ovaries to produce more eggs. Then multiple eggs (between 10 and 15 eggs) can be harvested in one procedure. Embryos withstand the **cryopreservation** process much better than eggs do.


## The Legacy of the Baby M Trial

On March 27, 1986, Mary Beth Whitehead, a 28-year-old White mother of two children, gave birth to a daughter whom she and her husband named Sara Elizabeth Whitehead. The baby was the biological daughter of Mary Beth Whitehead, a surrogate, and the biological child of William Stern, a 38-year-old biochemist. Ms. Whitehead had signed the surrogacy contract prior to being impregnated with the sperm of Mr. Stern. She had agreed to relinquish the child for adoption and give up her rights as the mother so that Mrs. Elizabeth Stern could adopt the child. She changed her mind after the birth and fought for custody. Prior to this high-profile custody battle, few Americans were aware of this technology and it was relatively uncommon. Because Mary Beth Whitehead had a genetic tie to the child and was the mother as well as the surrogate, there was ambiguity surrounding the issue of whether she could be forced to give up her maternal status. She had not yet signed the adoption papers so she was technically still the legal guardian. Her name and that of her husband were listed on the birth certificate.

When Ms. Whitehead refused to sign the adoption papers and relinquish her rights as the legal mother, a custody dispute ensued that would mesmerize the nation. Whitehead had signed a surrogacy contract with William and Elizabeth Stern in February of

1985. According to this agreement, in exchange for $10,000 she would surrender the baby to Mr. Stern and relinquish all parental rights thus allowing him to be adopted by Elizabeth Stern who had no genetic tie to the child. After giving birth and seeing her daughter Mary Beth Whitehead changed her mind and decided to keep the baby whom she breastfed for 40 days. A custody battle ensued and they went to court to fight for Sara Elizabeth, who was named Melissa Elizabeth Stern by the Sterns and became known as "Baby M" by the press. This case raised a number of issues involving surrogacy, contract law, parental rights, and ultimately led to the State of New Jersey banning commercial surrogacy. An analysis of the media coverage provides insights into the ways that class and power played out in the treatment of Mary Beth Whitehead. The judge granted custody to Mr. Stern but also allowed Mary Beth Whitehead to retain her material rights and gave her limited visitation privileges.

In 1987 the New Jersey Court ruled that surrogacy contracts are unenforceable and then awarded custody of Baby M to Mr. William Stern, her biological father and his wife Elizabeth Stern while giving limited visitation rights to Mary Beth Whitehead, who remained the legal mother. Unlike today, this case occurred in a period when the gestational surrogate was also the genetic mother. Since William Stern's wife was unable to carry a pregnancy to term and would not be able to bear a child to whom she had a genetic tie, and Mary Beth Whitehead already had two children, the court compromised. They supported one portion of the contract, which gave Mr. Stern custody, but they refused to allow his wife to have her name put on the birth certificate thus upholding Mary Beth Whitehead's legal status as the mother. In the decision handed down the judge wrote,

> We invalidate the surrogacy contract because it conflicts with the law and public policy of this State. While we recognize the depth of yearning of infertile couples to have their own children, we find payment of money to a "surrogate" mother illegal, perhaps criminal, and potentially degrading to women.
>
> (Willentz 1988, as quoted in Oliver 1989: 95)

*Note :* This case divided feminists into two camps. Feminists who supported a woman's right to rent out her womb or uterus as part of a contract supported the Sterns while those who argued that commercial surrogacy is a form of baby-selling that commodifies women and their bodies opposed this decision. Kelly Oliver criticizes the liberal framework used by the courts to conceal social inequalities. Oliver argues that "Within a liberal framework all people are considered equal with equal rights. They all operate autonomously and have the freedom to exercise their rights as long as they don't interfere with the rights of others. In this framework, the surrogacy contract is seen as an agreement between two or more equal partners" (Oliver 1989: 98–99).

In the decades since the Baby M case, gestational surrogacy has replaced what is called "traditional" surrogacy for most individuals contracting. Gestational surrogacy enables the **intended mother** or parent to sever the "genetic tie" between the birth mother and the infant. In other words it enables women and men who are the intended parents to retain their genetic tie to the child even though they do not gestate it. In the case of women whose eggs are too old or not viable for other reasons, they can purchase anonymous ova and still sever the tie between the gestational surrogate and the child so that the genetic tie occurs between a woman who does not carry the child and has merely sold her genetic material to the intended parents.

Innovations in biomedicine have dramatically increased the fertility treatments available and made it possible for women who have no genetic relations to the fetuses they carry to serve as surrogates, also referred to as "gestational carriers." The tie between genetics and gestation has been severed. This has radically transformed the experience of family formation for women and men with fertility problems, particularly the group between the ages of 35 and 45.

In *The Baby Business*, Deborah Spar, a former faculty member of the Harvard Business School, provides a comprehensive analysis of the economic, legal, and technological foundations of the commercial surrogacy market. In her summary of the debates in the 1980s Spar outlines the ideological divisions between opponents and supporters of commercial surrogacy:

> [S]upporters of surrogacy framed their arguments in terms of either parental desperation (those who turned to surrogacy had no other means of producing a much-wanted child) or the freedom to contract (if individuals were allowed to procreate and to contract, then surely they should be able to procreate under contract). These arguments played out in both academic and public forums, pitting market advocates against the defenders of women's rights. Interestingly, most feminists aligned with traditional conservatives in this debate, arguing that women's rights did not include the right to sell procreative services. More libertarian feminists, by contrast, sided with the more radical free marketers, insisting that freedom for women included the freedom to contract for labor, be it working in a factory or bearing a child.
>
> (Spar 2006: 77)

These arguments continue to be recycled and resurrected into today's media accounts and tabloid docudramas involving surrogacy. What is missing in most of these debates and media representations and what was disappointingly lacking in Spar's analysis is the role of race, racism, and class inequalities in structuring the market logics. Who can enter into these contracts as a commissioning parent? And why are Blacks, Hispanics, Latinos, and poor women overrepresented as gestational surrogates?

Control over one's reproductive labor remains a privilege rather than a right in the United States. Whether one is discussing access to abortion, contraception, or IVF fertility treatments, services related to the reproductive functions of women are highly stratified along racial, ethnic, class, and religious lines. In the United States assisted reproductive technologies are not accessible to the poor, working class, and many members of racial and ethnic minorities. Access to fertility treatments is available primarily to the wealthy, upper middle class, or those able and willing to borrow the money required. In other words, commercial surrogacy is limited to the economically privileged. (The price for the cost of hiring a gestational surrogate including the costs of IVF, legal, travel, gifts, and related expenses can range from $50,000–100,000 depending on the number of live births, experience of surrogate, and region.)

Spar's analysis, although an important intervention into this debate, is limited by its failure to consider carefully the ways that racial inequalities and class inequalities structure the surrogacy industry in the United States and abroad. Black feminists and critical race scholars have opposed commercial surrogacy and have expressed skepticism about the meaning of consumer "choice" and "free" markets in a nation whose early economy was built on enslaved labor and slave-produced crops (for example, cotton, sugar, rice, indigo, tobacco).

For almost 300 years women of African ancestry worked as slave laborers and produced children who were commodities in a stratified system. As the mothers of children who constituted a form of wealth for their owners (and sometimes their biological fathers) they did not possess what Dorothy Roberts call **reproductive liberty**. They did not have control over their reproductive labor. They could not choose when to have children, or how many children to bear, and their children were commodities that did not belong to them. Critics might argue that non-slave women during this same period (i.e. White women) also possessed limited, if any, control over their reproductive lives as married women due to the lack of availability of contraception; however, there was one difference. Children born to non-slave mothers were not commodities that generated wealth or could be traded and sold like livestock. Moreover, their fathers, who were often Europeans or European-Americans, did not have to acknowledge any genetic ties they might have to these children who were born under slavery.

The significance of the legacies of racialized slavery, class inequalities, and the exploitation of the reproductive labor of Black women is not considered in Spar's analysis. This inattention to race (and racism) is characteristic of much of the academic and media accounts of surrogacy. In striking contrast, the Black feminist legal scholars see U.S. slavery and the lack of reproductive liberty as having structured and continuing to structure the experiences of large segments of the U.S. population including poor White women, immigrant women and women of obvious African ancestry.

In the United States there are no federal laws regulating surrogacy. Consequently, in contrast to Israel there have been a small number of controversial and high-profile court cases involving surrogacy contract disputes. The federal government's failure to regulate this industry has left it up to individual states to regulate. Consequently we have a patchwork of laws and competing and contradictory legislation in the United States. Some states, such as Arizona and the District of Columbia, ban all commercial surrogacy contracts, while others ban payments but allow for services (Florida, Nevada, New York, New Hampshire, Virginia, Washington), while others like California have become interstate and international destinations of choice for couples wishing to purchase reproductive services and hire surrogates.

Imagine that you can hire someone to carry a pregnancy to term for around the cost of a mid-sized car. And you can be insured that the woman's medical condition is monitored during the entire pregnancy. You are relieved because she is receiving adequate nutrition and under continual medical supervision. There are no opportunities for your gestational surrogate to consume alcohol, use recreational drugs, or smoke. If you have donated the eggs and the sperm, then the child also has a genetic tie to you. In other words, it belongs to you "genetically" because the genetic material (ovum, sperm) belongs to you or a sibling.

In the first of a three-part series of reports, after outlining the systematic corruption and economic coercion in the adoption or what some called the "baby trade" in Guatemala, one of the poorest countries in the Americas, Karen Smith Rotabi reveals that demand for babies is so great and the supply so low that surrogacy is now replacing adoption.

> Desperately poor Guatemalan women will inevitably find themselves offered an opportunity to earn a wage to birth a baby in this dollar-a-day-nation … The financial payment for surrogacy in Guatemala is unclear but inter-country adoption experts estimate that some women earned approximately $1,500 for child relinquishment signatures in the old adoption system which amounts to just over $5 a day for a normal 280 day gestational period. For a woman of privilege in the United States looking for fertility alternatives, this is a bargain basement price, but extreme poverty is the only reason why any Guatemalan women would agree to such an arrangement.
>
> (Rotabi 2010)

Today a growing number of children enter families via surrogates and surrogacy contracts. These contracts are essentially pre-conception legal agreements in which a woman agrees to rent her womb to another individual or couple for the purpose of gestating a fetus to which she may or may not have a genetic tie. The majority of women who provide gestational services are poor or members of racial or ethnic minority groups.

On November 30, 2008 *The New York Times Magazine* published "Her Body, My Baby," a cover story by Alex Kucyznski in which she reports on her own experiences of hiring a gestational surrogate. The magazine cover shows Alex Kuczysnki standing next to a pregnant White woman. Inside the magazine the article is accompanied by a photograph of Alex Kuczynski, a White upper middle class woman holding her baby while a Black baby nurse stands behind her at attention. She is poised in front of her home in South Hampton, an elite residential enclave on Long Island. As a White, married, upper middle class, economically secure woman with fertility problems Kuczynski symbolically represents women who have the financial resources to purchase the reproductive services of a surrogate. Supporters of commercial surrogacy would argue that Kuczynski had suffered enough, deserved to become a mother and had the right to "assistance." Opponents of commercial surrogacy would argue that this is a form of "baby brokering" and that a capitalist culture in the United States has generated a cult of genetic entitlement that has trained upper middle class women who near the end of their childbearing clock to feel that they must have (and deserve) a child with whom they have genetic tie. In the past these women would have adopted a child.

This issue has divided public policy makers and legislators in the United States. The result is a patchwork of divergent regulatory regimes in which some states completely ban commercial surrogacy, while others allow surrogacy but restrict payments to a third party and yet other states like California are surrogacy-friendly and allow all forms of commercial surrogacy without restrictions. Some feminists have argued in support of commercial surrogacy because they argue that women have the right or "freedom" to enter into surrogacy contracts, while others have compared surrogacy to "sex work"—a form of denigrated labor that exploits poor women. We must understand the economic, legal, global, and racial context of these decisions. Women do not make decisions in isolation from factors that structure their options. Their class position, race, nationality, maternal status, marital status, and legal condition shape their ability to exercise agency. These structures shape what constitutes a desirable option.

The 1990s marked a period of rapid innovations in assistive reproductive technologies. These medical technologies further severed the ties between the intended parents and the birth mother, or what is now typically referred to as the "gestational carrier" or "gestational surrogate." Commercial surrogacy splits the function of the mother into three components: 1) genetic, 2) gestational (biological), and 3) social. Gillian Goslinga-Roy argues that these distinctions are not

> "stable" and have to be constantly enacted. For example, she notes that "The professional language of assisted reproduction firmly upholds these divisions [between genetic, biological and social]: surrogates are referred to as "carriers" or "womb donors" pointing to their instrumentality in the arrangement while "intended" or "recipient" couples are referred to as the genetic (a.k.a. "real") parents.
>
> (Goslinga-Roy 2000: 113)

1. **Gestational surrogate:** This is the most common form of commercial surrogacy today. A woman who gestates a fetus (allows herself to be impregnated and carries the pregnancy to term) but has no genetic tie to the child she births. She is not the "intended" parent but is a paid laborer working on a nine-month commercial contract. There is an **embryo transfer** and she carries a child of which she is not the biological mother. Higher-income infertile couples who can afford the costs of paying someone to be a gestational carrier contract with a surrogate. This form of commercial surrogacy is illegal in Australia, Canada, Egypt, Mexico, and most of Europe.
2. **Traditional surrogate:** The birth mother is both the "gestational" surrogate and the biological mother (contributes the genetic material—the ovum). Like a gestational surrogate she is selling her reproductive labor, that is, renting her womb out for a fee. In contrast to "gestational" surrogates she has a genetic tie to the child she is carrying. In traditional case law she is the legally recognized mother until she relinquishes the child for adoption.
3. **Intended mother:** This is the woman who, either alone or with a male or female partner, commissions the pregnancy and enters into a commercial contract with another woman who agrees to be implanted with an embryo that consists of her ovum or donated ovum. The "intended" mother is understood to be the "commissioning mother" and typically custody of the baby is turned over to her upon the birth. Her name, not the gestational surrogate's, is listed on the birth certificate.

Since 1997 private clinics have been required to report their IVF statistics to the Center for Disease Control. However, accurate national data does not exist about the number of *private* arrangements because birth certificates are not required to list how a baby came to be fertilized. In 2005 the Center for Disease Control recorded 1,012 gestational surrogacy/IVF surrogacy/IVF attempts using non-donor embryos (Center for Disease Control 2006: 3). In 2008 the Center for Disease Control published a national report on outcomes of their AVF cycles. According to the 2006 CDC National Report on Fertility 10 percent of the 62 million women of childbearing age in the United States have received some infertility services at some time in their lives (2006: 3–4).

## DISCUSSION QUESTIONS

1. If your sister, friend, or family member learned that she was not able to carry a pregnancy to term, would you support her hiring a gestational surrogate? What would your arguments in support of/against it be?
2. Should assisted reproductive technologies be sold by profit-making companies or should they be provided free of charge and paid for as part of a health insurance plan?
3. Should the fertility industry be regulated by the federal government so that we have uniform laws in each state? Today individuals who live in some states have access to this legally while in other states it is banned or criminalized so they would have to travel to a different state to purchase these services if their state doesn't permit it.

# II: Racism, Capitalism, and Reproductive Labor

～～✕～～

Before the advent of the assisted reproductive technologies employed today, older forms of surrogacy were used. There are biblical examples from Genesis (Chapter 30) in which Rachel, who is infertile, gives Bilhah, her servant (or slave) to Jacob as a concubine to serve as a surrogate. Bilhah gives birth to two sons whom Rachel names and considers her children. This is the earliest biblical example of what could be called surrogate mothers. As servants and concubines with no rights, these women had little power and seemed to have no control over their bodies or their reproductive labor, which could be used by their mistresses and the patriarchs for whom they served as surrogates. They were used to conceive a child that was genetically related to the father. These women, like U.S. slaves, were not recognized as the legal mothers of their children.

In Europe there was another tradition that Deborah Spar describes as an earlier form of surrogacy.

> Another form of surrogacy arose in the Middle Ages, when wealthy women regularly turned their newborns over to wet nurses: nursing mothers who, for a fee, would assume the care and feeding of an additional child. Typically the child would live with the wet nurse during the first year of life, with the mother making only occasional visits. In many respects, this relationship is the closest antecedent to modern-day commercial surrogacy. The surrogate generally has no long-term involvement with the child; she is employed for a specific task and paid a nontrivial fee. The surrogate tends to be poorer then the mothers they serve and to have their own biological children. *(sic)*

(Spar 2006: 73)

A historical and comparative analysis of the experiences of enslaved women can illuminate how capitalism and racism restricted the reproductive liberty of Black women for hundreds of years. In this section, we will consider how U.S.-born Blacks (who were often of European ancestry also) have been denied reproductive liberty and the implications of this for ethical debates about the ethical treatment of gestational surrogates.

Who is allowed or encouraged to procreate and under what conditions? An analysis of the meaning of reproductive liberty illuminates how power asymmetries operate and how structural inequalities are reinforced and socially reproduced. Between the 17th century and the latter half of the 19th century, the wombs of Black women and all enslaved women of multiracial heritage in the United States and other slave-holding societies in the Americas and the Caribbean were treated as commercial surrogates. They were expected to produce children for men to whom they were not married and they had no legal rights to their birth children. Their children were commodities that were bought and sold on the market. Racialized slavery structured the reproductive lives of millions of women and was a form of **forced surrogacy**.

## U.S. Slavery and the Historical Commodification of Reproduction

Black feminist legal theorists have drawn several parallels between the exploitation of Black women's reproductive labor during and after slavery and that of contemporary surrogates. For example, Anita Allen, a U.S. Black feminist legal scholar argues that the use of Black surrogates is an extension of historical racial and class hierarchies that controlled the reproductive division of labor for several hundred years prior to emancipation. This is a historical case of commodified reproduction upon which the U.S. economy was based. In the words of Allen,

> Commercial surrogacy encourages society to think of economically and socially vulnerable women as disposable for a price. Segments of the public will draw the obvious parallels to slavery and prostitution. Their reaction may seem melodramatic. But it is a telling reminder of social attitudes and history.
>
> (Allen 1991: 30)

> The American slave experience, while not equivalent to the surrogate, can help illuminate why many people find the practice of commercial surrogacy disturbing. Before the American Civil War, virtually all southern Black women were, in a sense, surrogate mothers. Slave women knowingly gave birth to children with the understanding that these children would be owned by others. The fear among black feminists is that poor women and black women in particular could become a "surrogate class" for affluent white women and other economically privileged women.
>
> (Allen 1991: 17)

Black feminists who have argued in favor of criminalizing commercial surrogacy contracts focus on the unique vulnerabilities of Black surrogates who have been neglected in most analyses (Allen 1991). The commodification of babies and their sale have their roots in the capitalist system of slavery in the United States. In a rare analysis of the surrogacy system, Cheryl J. Sanders argues that the American slave system was based on "forced surrogacy."

The system of racial slavery established in the United States forced enslaved women of African ancestry who had no social, political, or economic rights to give birth to generations of children who were commodities. As slaves their children were "owned" by other people.

Although contemporary gestational surrogates "voluntarily" enter into these commercial contracts and willingly sell their "reproductive" labor, their agency occurs within a context of a stratified system of reproduction. Kelly Oliver reminds us that commercial surrogacy occurs within a capitalist system in which market forces constrain the choices of poor women and that

> Most people do not perform their services 24 hours a day unless they are slaves. And most people only sell their labor, labor performed by the body, perhaps but distinguishable from it. Surrogates, on the other hand, perform their services 24 hours a day and sell the body itself … She is never off-duty.

(1989: 97–98)

## Commercial Surrogacy as a Form of Stratified Contract Labor

Surrogacy is a form of **commercial or contract labor** that involves purchasing the "reproductive labor" of a third party in order to conceive and bring to term a baby. It includes in vitro fertilization, embryo transfers, and other forms of assisted reproduction. This form of labor involves the purchase and sale or rental of the bodily functions of a woman and the child that results from this labor in exchange for payment. Surrogacy is a gender-specific form of industrial labor. Surrogacy has been described by feminist opponents as "the industrialization of pregnancy" and as a "degradation" of women's reproductive labor. Despite the altruistic motives that may inspire some women to serve as gestational surrogates, this is a form of contract labor that involves physical risks, pain, and possible death, as well as invasive medical procedures.

Commercial surrogacy is severely restricted or banned in most industrialized nations. Most industrialized nations including Australia, Canada, China, the Czech Republic, Denmark, France, Germany, Italy, Mexico, Taiwan, Turkey, and several U.S. States ban surrogacy. The United Kingdom, Brazil, and Israel have partial bans.

Legal scholars opposed to commercial surrogacy have argued that commercial surrogacy or **"contract pregnancy"** can best be conceptualized as a form of "estranged labor." Kelly Oliver uses the concept of "estranged labor" to argue that the liberal framework employed by U.S. judges conceals the class inequalities and gender hierarchies that will guarantee that surrogates lose custody of their child (1989). Drawing on Marx's distinction between estranged and alienated labor, Oliver shows how the judicial use of a liberal framework disempowers surrogates. She argues that "Using the jargon of rights, the liberal framework conceals social and class interests behind the illusion of formal equality in contracts" (Oliver 1989: 96).

Others have argued that this is not the case and that some mothers do not experience alienation (Teman 2010). Later we will see that the national and religious context can structure the emotional experience of gestational surrogates and that some women may not experience it as "estranged" labor while others might. The data thus far is not conclusive on this issue.

The economic benefits of motherhood are structured along racial, ethnic, and class lines with poor women renting their wombs out for service to higher-income women and couples in exchange for capital. They are selling their bodily labor, to more economically privileged women. Surrogacy is an industry that is embedded in racial and class hierarchies. Commercial surrogacy can best be understood as a form of stratified reproduction in which poor women and increasingly women from racial and ethnic backgrounds are renting their wombs out or "selling their uterus" to wealthier women and men in exchange. They lack the economic, social, and cultural resources of the couple whom they serve. Yet White surrogates remain advantaged over Blacks in that they can always refuse to accept work from Black couples seeking a surrogate. They can (and do) practice racial exclusions. The ongoing racial discrimination in the labor market, and the fact that Blacks have a higher poverty rate than Whites, means Black surrogates are less likely to refuse work.

In U.S. policy debates for or against surrogacy there has been insufficient analytical attention given to the role that economic privilege plays in access to ART and whether this form of inequality should be supported. With a few notable exceptions U.S. public policy debates about the ethics of commercial surrogacy have been framed in ways that avoid obvious histories of the commodification of slave children and the contemporary commodification of White children. In an analysis of the competing frames of surrogacy, Susan Markens identifies the frames and concludes that "the analysis also shows how those advocates both for and against commercial surrogacy shared many fundamental assumptions about the nature of the family and were similarly blind to the significant disparities between racial/ethnic groups' real access to procreative rights" (2007: 81). In striking contrast to the analysis offered by non-Blacks in surrogacy debates, Markens acknowledges that these frames reflect the priorities and racialized concerns of affluent White women.

Supporters of commercial surrogacy argue that women have the right to enter into these commercial contracts and that this form of what Chesler referred to as "industrial pregnancy" is not worse than other forms of labor and provides more income for less work. Mothers can stay at home with their birth children and take care of them, or pay for their education while assisting others in achieving their goal of becoming parents. Supporters or proponents of commercial surrogacy emphasize that this is "voluntary" and that these women are not forced to enter into this agreements. They stress the advantages and benefits of this job compared to other work. However, the issue of "voluntary" labor must be understood in the context of the job market and the absence of living wage jobs for many women without a college education.

In India, commercial surrogacy was legalized in 2002. Since that time, India has quickly emerged as an international magnet for surrogacy services due to the high quality of the medical clinics, the supervision of the gestational surrogates and the low cost relative to the United States and Europe. There are no comprehensive laws regulating surrogacy. A draft law called the Assisted Reproductive Technology (Regulation) Bill 2008 was ready for parliamentary ratification in 2009. Anoop Gupta, a Delhi fertility doctor, says, "Surrogacy is the new adoption." Surrogacy is estimated to be a $445 million business in India, where the costs of treatment are comparatively low compared with the United States and Europe. The Confederation of Indian Industry predicts that medical tourism, including surrogacy, could generate $2.3 billion in annual revenue by 2012. Gestational surrogacy is an important gendered niche in the global medical market.

One of the largest clinics in India is the Akanksha Infertility Clinic run by Dr. Nayana Patel and her husband. Since 2003, 167 surrogate mothers have successfully given birth to 216 babies at this clinic. This clinic has been the subject of numerous media reports and is seen as one of the main hubs of the Indian global surrogacy market. A journalistic account of gestational surrogacy in India was published in *Mother Jones* in 2010. In this article Scott Carney reports,

> In exchange for the inconvenience and physical discomforts, they stand to receive a sum that's quite substantial by their meager standards, but which the clinic's customers understand is a steal. The customers are mostly foreigners—three of the city's boarding houses are constantly booked with American, British, French, Japanese and Israeli surrogacy tourists.

> (Carney 2010: 70)

Although these surrogates can earn as much as $5,000–6,000 if they do not have a miscarriage this is a fraction of what it would cost to pay for these same services in the United States, where the costs could range between $50,000–120,000 with medical and legal fees. One criticism of this clinic is that the women are primarily from very poor and rural backgrounds with most being barely literate.

There is a paradox here that is often neglected in media accounts of these Indian clinics. Women who become gestational surrogates in India live in a country which has the highest maternal mortality rate in South Asia after Bangladesh. The rate of death is 301 in 100,000 births (World Bank). Moreover the rate of illiteracy for girls is high, and educational opportunities are structured by caste hierarchies. In India gestational surrogacy may be the only attractive option for many women who seek to supplement their husband's income. However, these women, like their U.S. counterparts, are exercising a form of constrained agency since their options are severely limited by caste hierarchies, class inequality, limited education, and legal regimes that may not regulate this industry. The coercive aspect of this form of commercial labor is masked by the fact that the alternatives are working for 10–15 years to earn an equivalent income. The income inequality and the fact that women with alternatives are not entering this labor niche tend to be minimized in the media representations.

## The U.S. Labor Market: Constrained Occupational Choices

The market for commercial surrogates, **egg donors**, sperm donors, and other forms of assisted reproduction has expanded rapidly during the past two decades. The labor market does not provide statistics specifically on the participation of women and men in this market. In part, it is difficult to track because individuals who sell their genetic material often do it for short periods of time and often to a private agency so they may or may not report this income. Moreover, private arrangements regarding gestational surrogates would not be tracked by the U.S. Department of Labor. Because this industry remains unregulated at the federal level and the state regulations vary by state, there is no database that provides statistics on the race, class, gender, and number of surrogates participating at any given moment in this industry.

In order to understand surrogacy as a market, let's compare the occupations and income levels in which U.S. women aged 16 and older are concentrated. This enables us to see the employment options that are available for women who seek to become gestational surrogates. The average income for gestational surrogate varies by her experience, region of the country, and whether she gives birth to singletons or twins. For a single birth, the pay ranges between $20,000 and $25,000, not including any after-birth cash gifts.

In 2009 the U.S. Department of Labor reported that 72 million women age 16 years or older were participating in the labor market. This constitutes 59.2 percent of the 122 million women in this age group who were actively seeking work or employed. Women who were not employed professionals were concentrated in the following job categories: personal care and service occupations, and sales and office occupations.

How do the wages of a gestational surrogate compare with that of women working in other industries that provide comparable pay? A brief analysis of the Department of Labor statistics for employed women reveals which job categories provide a comparable wage. Occupations are structured by gender so only 1 percent of women could be found in occupations in the natural resources, construction, and maintenance fields. Women were concentrated in jobs that involved service, personal care, and professional. Listed below are the largest occupational categories for female workers in 2009.

1. Secretaries and administrative assistants.
2. Registered nurses.
3. Elementary and middle school teachers.
4. Cashiers.
5. Nursing, psychiatric and home health aides.
6. Retail salespersons.
7. First-line managers of retail sales workers.
8. Waiters and waitresses.
9. Maids and housekeeping cleaners.
10. Customer service representatives.
11. Child care workers.

Under the category of personal care and service occupations, those jobs that were closest to the wages of a surrogate included:

- Nursing home health aides $24,010.
- Personal and home care aides $20,110.
- Hairdresser, hair stylists $22,580.
- Medical records clerks $28,870.
- Cashiers $18,650.
- Counter and retail clerks $20,870.
- Retail sales persons $24,570.

We can see that for carrying a pregnancy to term a gestational surrogate can earn as much as or more than the median income for a woman working in retail sales or as a nursing or home health aide. This enables her to be a stay-at-home worker while carrying for her children. It is also an extension of her childcaring and maternal duties and therefore does not challenge the gendered hierarchies in the labor force or call attention to what Arlie Hochschild (2003) calls the "**second shift**," in which employed women return home and do another shift of domestic work. In addition, surrogates can receive medical benefits and often a monthly stipend if they are not already insured. This may be perceived as an attractive alternative to working in jobs that provide comparable wages, especially for women who are the mothers of young children, the wives of active duty military or who have neither the time nor economic resources to return to school to obtain an advanced degree or professional training required to become a licensed nurse or occupational therapist, which are two of the highest paid occupations for women, with an annual median income of $60,540.

Class inequalities, the legacies of racial slavery, and gender segregation in the labor market structure the global surrogacy industry. Proponents of commercial surrogacy describe this form of reproductive service work as a "choice." The sale of sex-specific reproductive labor is made to appear as "natural." The question of how economic coercion is concealed within a discourse of "choice" and rights remains unanswered.

## DISCUSSION QUESTIONS

1. How would you define reproductive liberty?
2. Do poor women really have reproductive liberty if they can't afford to pay for health care, including getting an abortion if they wish to terminate a pregnancy?
3. Do you support a woman's right to rent out her body as a surrogate? Explain why you oppose or support this form of contract labor.
4. How does commercial surrogacy differ from other forms of labor?

# III:  Becoming a Gestational Surrogate

〜✕〜

Y̲ou would like to earn some fast cash. You are a full-time homemaker and the mother of one or two children. You are married. You would like to supplement your family's income to pay for a vacation, your children's education, save for a room addition, pay for tutoring for a child who has special needs, or pay off debt. You may be employed but would like to supplement your income to pay for unusual expenses. You have a child who has special medical needs and you want to convert your basement into a physical therapy gym for your child. You want to have a financial cushion because although your spouse or domestic partner is employed, he earns a modest income that doesn't cover all of the household needs. In other words, you are working class or middle class and financially challenged.

You can go on the Internet and find out which surrogacy agencies are recruiting surrogates in your region. If you are fortunate and live in a highly competitive market such as southern California or parts of the Northeast where there is a concentration of agencies who are competing for surrogates, this will increase the potential fees. You can either register with an agency or you can place your own advertisement on craigslist indicating that you are available. Placing your own advertisement gives you more control over whom you sell your reproductive services to in this market.

Three recruitment advertisements by surrogacy agencies from the Northeast, one from California's Central Coast, and another from Los Angeles illustrate the wages available and the type of language used by these agencies to present gestational surrogacy as a safe and easy way to make fast cash.

---

**Massachusetts**

*Boston craigslist: The Center for Surrogacy and Egg Donation, Inc.*

SUBJECT HEADING: SURROGATE MOTHER NEEDED—HELP A COUPLE HAVE A CHILD, EARN $35K PLUS (BOSTON AND SURROUNDING AREAS)

- Earn between $20,000 and $25,000 for a first-time surrogacy, and significantly more as an experienced surrogate.
- Enjoy the financial freedom of being able to pay off your student loan, make a down payment on a home, or create a college fund for your own children.
- Retain 100% of your fee, as all expenses will be paid through our agency.

---

What we see from these recruitment advertisements is that the discomfort, health risks and any potential medical dangers are not explicitly mentioned or addressed. There is also a tension between emphasizing the "fast cash" while also stating that the potential surrogate must be financially independent.

## Independent Advertisements by Surrogates

Some surrogates place their own advertisements on the Internet. This gives them more control over whose child they would carry. They can represent themselves without having to conform to the constraints of the agencies, which may have non-discrimination policies. For example, some prospective surrogates may hold strong religious beliefs and may not want to carry a child for same sex couples or for individuals who are not Christians. Here are some examples of how surrogates represent themselves as "free agents."

> I am a non-religious 35-year-old happily married mother of three (7½, 4, 17 months) who wants to help you realize your dream of being a parent. I have had 3 full-term pregnancies with no complications.

Within the gestational surrogacy market, a niche has emerged for surrogates willing to carry babies to term for same sex couples. Agencies such as SurrogateAlternatives.com advertise to same sex couples seeking a surrogate. The website for Surrogate Alternatives targets gays and lesbians. Their website reaches out to same sex couples with reassurance and emphasizes the legal support that they offer and the changes in attitudes. For example:

> Years ago being gay meant a living a life without children. Never being able to hold or love a child that is biologically your own. That has all changed!!! You are no longer restricted due to your sexuality and people aren't as closed minded about men raising children without a mother in the dynamic ... This medical procedure allows for BOTH parents to fertilize the embryo and to transfer one embryo fertilized by one parents and the second fertilized by the other, thus if both embryos grow into the babies, the clients would know each has a biological child on the way.

Sometimes single gay men post their own adverts for surrogates while working with an attorneys who specialize in surrogacy. These men tend to be well-paid professionals who are seeking a surrogate because they do not have a sibling or close female friend who can serve as a surrogate for them. In other words, they do not have access to an altruistic surrogate within their familial or friendship network. Like heterosexual couples they use the sperm of the husband/intended father and purchase the ovum; they are splitting the function between the donor (genetic mother) and the carrier (gestational surrogate), which also minimizes legal problems since the gestational surrogate who gives birth to the child has no genetic tie to the child she carries. An example of an advertisement posted in the summer of 2010 on craigslist represents the approach of single gay men.

This ad also shows the market value of experience. Having previously carried a pregnancy to term and given birth as a gestational surrogate increases one's market value and the wages that one can command because it demonstrates that a woman is already familiar with the process and has delivered a desirable product. Depending upon the region, wealth, and desperation of the contracting person, this experience can translate into an additional $5,000–10,000 in wages. Another factor, however, is the number of available (and acceptable) surrogates in a region. In a competitive region where agencies and intended parents are competing for the most desirable surrogates, the price that a surrogate can command (as well as an egg donor) increases.

### Racism Among U.S. Gestational Surrogates: A San Francisco Case

Social inequalities and racial hierarchies were exacerbated by breaking the genetic tie; women from racial and ethnic minorities can now bear children for women from high-income and racially dominant groups—thus extending a long history of poor women and women of color doing a form of service work and nurturing labor—modern-day "wet nurses."

In her research in the San Francisco Bay area, Goslinga-Roy found that "race" or Blackness was a significant factor in how the White gestational surrogate she followed during the entire process maintained her bodily integrity. She uncovered racist ideologies that structured her experience of the surrogacy process. Some White surrogates refuse to gestate a child that is the product of Black parents. According to Goslinga-Roy's analysis the absolute rejection of Blacks and refusal to serve as a gestational surrogate for a Black couple enabled this White surrogate to maintain a feeling of bodily integrity. She notes that "Julie" explained that:

> It feels foreign to me. Different. I could carry a Japanese baby or a Chinese baby because they are white to me. Society sees them as white. But a Black child is more difficult. I'm already surrounded by controversy: I married a man thirty-two years older than me. I work in a later-term, problem-pregnancy abortion facility, and I'm a surrogate. To give birth to a Black child would add one more controversial aspect to my life and I'm not ready to be on the front page of the National Enquirer.

> (Goslinga-Roy 2000: 116)

In her analysis of this quote, Goslinga-Roy argues that,

> What struck me more, however, was how carrying *someone else's* (White) child provoked no gut reaction in her whatsoever ... But the mere thought of carrying someone else's *Black* child immediately made her experience of surrogacy as a very intimate and at once very public violation of her bodily and moral boundaries. Whiteness, I had to conclude, was the invisible glue that held her narrative of gestational surrogacy together.

> (Goslinga-Roy 2000: 116)

Technological innovations have allowed people to select surrogates who are classified as "racially" different from them to carry their fetus because there is no "genetic" tie, thus it is simply a form of "labor." During the past decades there has been a dramatic change in the fertility industry among higher-income people primarily of European, European-American, Canadian, and Asian backgrounds selecting surrogates from a racial, ethnic, or national group presumed to be different from their own. Helena Ragoné identified a preference emerging in which a segment of the market expresses a preference for gestational surrogates who they perceive as racially or ethnically different from themselves (2000). In the aftermath of the Calvert trial, some argue that this is an attempt by intended parents to minimize the possibility of legal conflicts over infants born under surrogacy contracts.

In her analysis of the *shifting* and paradoxical meaning of the genetic tie, Dorothy Roberts argues that

> The institution of slavery made the genetic tie to the slave mother critical to determining a child's social status, yet legally insignificant to the relationship between male slave owners and their mulatto children. Although today we generally assume that the genetic tie creates an enduring bond between parents and their children,

the law often disregards it in the cases of surrogate mothers, sperm donors and unwed fathers.

(Roberts 1995: 210–11)

## Body Maps and Boundary Maintenance: The Israeli Experience

How do gestational surrogates experience the process of contract motherhood? How do they manage interpersonal boundaries? In *Birthing a Mother: The Surrogate Body and the Pregnant Self*, Elly Teman provides rare insights into this experience from the perspective of Israeli gestational surrogates and their intended mothers. From Teman we learn how gestational surrogates manage their interpersonal boundaries as contract laborers with the intended mother.

Israel is distinct for being the first and only country in the world that allows and funds surrogacy but regulates it in accordance with religious law at the state level. The surrogacy market in Israel is an internal market, in that it is restricted to Israeli citizens. Israeli gestational surrogates are only allowed to work for Israeli citizens. The Israeli government does not support or encourage reproductive tourism for heterosexual couples or unmarried women.

All surrogacy contracts must be pre-approved by a screening committee in advance. Israel has a set of strict criteria that is applied to all couples seeking a state-funded support for in vitro fertilization and surrogacy. Couples must be Israeli citizens or permanent residents, which prevents Israel from becoming a global commercial destination for **surrogacy tourism**. Couples seeking surrogates are also religiously matched to a gestational surrogate, which means that no Muslims and few Christian Arabs have participated in or have access to gestational surrogates.

Lesbians and unmarried Jewish women in Israel have access to services that are denied to gay men. Same sex lesbian couples can provide their own eggs and are allowed to purchase sperm and utilize IVF services that are state funded while same sex Israeli male couples are not given access to IVF services or to surrogates. While the Aloni Commission gave women, regardless of marital status, the right to become parents, this same right was not extended to unmarried men. Same sex couples that involve gay men must seek ART outside of Israel because they are not able to secure approval from a state committee to use ART. Thus, while lesbians or unmarried heterosexual women can form families with the support of the Israeli government, these services are not available to gay men, who must purchase procreative material and services outside of Israel. Gay men in Israel are a neglected market and like their U.S. and European counterparts, they become reproductive tourists, and travel to the United States or India to purchase ART services and to hire a gestational surrogate.

In the summer of 2010, a documentary produced by an Israeli filmmaker, titled *Google Baby*, was distributed by HBO cable television. In this film we meet several gay Israeli men who are seeking women from whom to purchase eggs and gestational surrogates. We move from the U.S. to India as we follow the process of selecting and buying and selling genetic material and ultimately acquiring a baby that was gestated by a woman in India.

When we compare the typical profile of a U.S. surrogate to that of an Israeli surrogate we find several differences that are notable. First, the average age of an Israeli surrogate is older. This is legislated by the Approval Committee. They must be:

- Unmarried.
- Must be recognized as Jewish.
- Older than 22 and younger than 40 years.
- Have given birth to at least one child.
- Have not given birth more than five times.
- Have not had more than two Cesarean sections.

In addition to the above characteristics women can be rejected as potential surrogates if they are:

- Obese.
- Have taken antidepressants.
- Have a history of smoking.

How do gestational surrogates manage their bodily integrity and create a zone of privacy for themselves while undergoing "invasive" medical procedures? In Emily Teman's (2010) groundbreaking ethnographic analysis of Jewish Israeli surrogates she uncovered several strategies that they employed to create a private zone on their body.

Elly Teman found that Israel surrogates use **body maps** in order to distance themselves from the fetuses that they are carrying and to manage interpersonal boundaries between themselves and the contracting couples. A body map is a conceptual tool used to inscribe symbolic lines of demarcation on their bodies. According to Teman:

> This enables gestational surrogates to distinguish between parts of the body they wish to personalize and parts they wish to distance, both cognitively and emotionally. On the basis of body maps, the women conceptually divide their bodies into different parts that they view as varyingly detached or connected to their own body and to their intended mother's body. Surrogates use the body map to form an interlinked, networked connection with their intended mother for the duration of the pregnancy.

> (Teman 2010: 25)

In Israel, in contrast to the U.S. and India, there is an absence of the racial and ethnic differences and religious difference that characterize many, if not most, surrogate-intended parent relationships. Surrogates are not racially or religiously matched in the U.S. (although racial matching may be the norm in terms of egg and sperm donors). The religious and ethnic matching of surrogates to the intended parents required by the Israeli screening committee contributes to an experience that may mitigate against the forms of alienation or "estranged" labor that has been suggested by U.S. analysts. However, to date there are no comparable sociological studies based on U.S. data that draw upon years of participant observation and the ethnographic relationships that Teman developed over an eight-year period. More studies are needed that can provide insights into how women located in different national, religious, cultural, and economic contexts conceptualize and experience their bodies.

Teman also identified a number of strategies employed by the Israeli Jewish gestational surrogates to shift their pregnant body symbolically to the intended mother. The Israeli surrogates and their intended mothers (contracting couples) engaged in practices that increased physical intimacy and dissolved the boundaries between the pregnant body of the surrogate and the non-pregnant body of the intended mother. For example, Teman found that "Women often used coupling and marriage imagery to describe their connection" (Teman 2010: 161). These intimacy strategies were designed to shift the experience of pregnancy to the intended mother thus creating the experience of a vicarious pregnancy:

- Mutual abstinence from sexual intercourse with boyfriends or husbands.
- Sleeping together in the marital bed.
- Intended mother will hold and caress the belly of the surrogate for extended periods of time.
- Public display of kissing and hugging.
- Surrogate and intended mother will hold hands and express affection in public.
- Intended mother administers hormone injections into the buttocks of the surrogate.

These intimacy strategies enable the gestational surrogate and the intended mother to merge their bodies and to shift the embodied experience—that is, the pregnant body to the intended mother who is not pregnant. In Israel, like the United States, genetics is privileged over gestation and according to Teman "environmental factors such as nutrition, overall care, weight gain and rest are downplayed in this interpretative model." Gestational surrogates use the Hebrew word **pundekaut**, which means "innkeeper," to describe their contribution as carriers, which minimizes the womb (and the surrogate's blood) as a significant environment in the development of the fetus.

## DISCUSSION QUESTIONS

1. Go online and review ten advertisements placed by surrogates. Based on your review, what is the primary motivation for women to rent themselves out as surrogates?

2. Should gestational surrogates have the right to discriminate against recipients of their services on the basis of race if they have already agreed to carry a child for someone of a different racial or ethnic background?

3. What do you see as the benefits and disadvantages of a gestational surrogate having a close relationship with the intended mother? Do you think it makes it harder for the surrogate to separate from the intended mother after the birth?

4. There is more social equality between Israeli gestational surrogates and the intended mother compared with the United States. Do you think that racial, ethnic, and religious matching of gestational surrogates and the intended parents would be more fulfilling for U.S. surrogates?

# IV:   Google Babies

## Class, Colorism, and Consumer Culture

~~~

You have not become pregnant after more than 24 months of engaging in unprotected sex with your husband or partner. You have decided not to adopt because you and/or your partner want to have a child who is genetically related. You are in a same sex relationship and neither you nor your male partner can give birth so you need to hire a gestational surrogate. What do you do? You go to your computer, type in "I want to get pregnant.com" or do a Google search. Your online search gives you access to a database of national and international infertility centers and surrogacy agencies.

Today it is relatively easy to use the Internet to research and identify agencies that will provide one-stop shopping for assistance in conception including the purchase of genetic material (ova, sperm) and to find a surrogate to hire. For example, www.iwanttogetpregnant.com is a website that offers services in India. The Internet now provides access to online shopping for a surrogate—an international database of women who will sell their ova or their reproductive services. This is a radical change in the consumption of fertilily services. According to Morgan,

> One of the most remarkable developments affecting surrogacy since it achieved public visibility has been the use of the Internet. It is used to search for and to advertise surrogacy services; to provide information about services; and to record surrogates' and intended parents' own stories about surrogacy arrangements. One of the main uses of the internet for these purposes is to enable people to circumvent domestic legal regimes that are either hostile to or prohibit surrogacy; the Internet is a passport for those who would wish to surf as a "procreative tourist."
>
> (Morgan 2003: 88)

You are affluent enough to travel to another state or another country to purchase the services of a gestational surrogate. But you want the highest "quality" product for the cheapest price. Where do you go? Affluent women in Asia, the Middle East, Europe, and the Americas routinely travel to the United States (and increasingly India which now offers them a "better deal"—a baby at the fraction of the cost). If surrogacy is banned in your state or country, you can travel to a surrogate-friendly state such as

California. This is called reproductive tourism. In other words, it is possible to avoid the regulatory regimes in one's own state, region, or nation. Women and men who live in Austria, Egypt, France, Italy, Mexico, Germany, Japan, Norway, the Netherlands, Spain, Sweden, and Switzerland cannot enter into surrogacy contracts, which are banned. Some U.S. states and European countries ban payments to surrogates. And many countries in most of Asia and Africa have no regulations regarding surrogacy because there is no industry and no facilities. Individuals who live in countries where either surrogacy is banned or payments to third parties are banned can travel to other nations to purchase these services. These regional disparities are combined with racial, ethnic, religious, and class gaps, which produce power inequities between the intended or commissioning parent(s) and the gestational (surrogate) mother.

Agencies advertise for surrogates online. The classified advertisements that recruit surrogates and the advertisements that potential surrogates place provide some insights into this industry. Here is a sample of what an American shopping for fertility services will find on the Internet. An online advertisement from The Surrogacy Advantage emphasizes the difference in the legal landscape in Illinois compared with other states where commercial surrogacy is prohibited.

> Unlike many states in which surrogate agreements are illegal or unenforceable, Illinois law allows intended parents to enter into legally enforceable agreements, providing security and legal protections for all parties involved. Illinois also provides an opportunity for intended parents to be recognized as a child's legal parents from the moment that child is born without an adoption or court proceedings as long as at least one of the parents is the genetic parent of that child.
>
> (http://www.egg411.com/SurrogacyAdvantage.html)

Like other full-service or one-stop agencies, The Surrogacy Advantage offers surrogacy health insurance contracts, provision of lodgings for out-of-state surrogates and their families, referral to a legal specialist, referrals for psychological testing, nutrition counselor for the surrogate as well as insured and bonded escrow services to handle the payments.

The typical profile of a U.S. surrogate (Center for Surrogate Parenting) is:

- Married.
- 21–37 years old.
- Has given birth to two children.
- 13 years of formal education.
- Stay-at-home mother.
- Economically vulnerable due to her dependency upon her husband's income.
- If employed, salary is not sufficient to achieve middle class status.

Research by cultural anthropologists has shown that consumers and ART agencies that supply genetic material employ racial logics and place higher value on genetic material provided by classified as/or presumed to be Whites. Consumers (particularly those who do not self-identify as Black) typically associate lighter skin and whiteness with desirability. These relationships are structured by racial and class inequality. Proponents of surrogacy employ the rhetoric of consumer rights and consumer choice while ignoring the practices of economic coercion, folklore beliefs in White racial purity, and skin color hierarchies that structure the fertility industry.

## Class, Colorism, and Consumer Choice in the Egg and Sperm Market

Single gay men, male couples, or heterosexual couples in which the woman's eggs are too old or otherwise compromised must purchase eggs as one stage in the process before or in conjunction with hiring a gestational surrogate. In many cases, the ovum is purchased from a woman who is not going to serve as the gestational surrogate. Twenty years ago, in what is now called traditional surrogacy, the woman who served as the gestational surrogate was also the genetic mother because she provided the ovum. With advances in assisted reproductive technologies this has become less common, especially for heterosexual couples. The commercial market in eggs and sperm has changed dramatically during the past two decades. This is a global market in which individuals can purchase ova or sperm from individuals in their own country, or in the case of Japan, France, Italy, Canada or places where this is banned, they can purchase it from elsewhere—say the United States or India. The terms **egg and sperm donation** are misnomers since individuals are not "donating" their eggs or sperm in an act of altruism, but selling them for a price.

Rene Lynn Almeling, a sociologist, conducted a rigorous study of the egg and sperm commercial market. Almeling provides an analysis of the way the sperm and egg market is organized to reinforce assumptions about gender roles and ideologies. Almeling also describes structural changes in this industry. In the late 1980s "physicians began to cede control of this process to commercial donation programs" and the "provision of gametes became the province of commercial agencies, rather than of medical professionals who first administered these technologies" (Almeling 2008: 38).

We learn from Almeling that class, education, gender, and sexual orientation play a role in the valuation of eggs. For example, based upon interviews with the directors of the largest commercial egg agencies, Almeling learns that in the United States, which is a relatively unregulated market, the fees that egg donors are paid vary according to their experience and their level of education, with first-time egg donors earning the least ($4,000) and experienced and well-educated egg donors earning substantially more ($6,000). Geographical location also played a role; in areas such as Los Angeles county there was stiff competition among commercial egg agencies who were aggressively competing for the eggs of desirable donors because they needed to maintain a diverse pool of donors (Almeling 2008: 95). Ameling found that race, class, and sexual orientation play a role in the valuation of the eggs, "due to the difficulty in maintaining a diverse pool of donors, both egg agencies often increase the fee for donors of color." Because so few Blacks can afford to hire gestational surrogates and they are excluded from the market due to poverty, some donors of color can command higher fees. In the case of recipients who may be wealthy and wish to purchase eggs, she notes that,

> If recipients are perceived as wealthy, the staff will often ask for a higher donor fee, as when an assistant mentions that "gay men, and single men have a lot of money, and they think nothing of seven, eight thousand dollars." ... If recipients experience a "failed cycle" with an egg agency's donor, the staff might offer a discounted rate on the second cycle.

> (Almeling 2008: 95)

Furthermore, in an analysis of the motivations that inspired women to sell their eggs, she found that financial incentives, rather than altruism, were often primary despite the corporate rhetoric of the "gift." In an analysis of the 19 egg donors interviewed, Almeling found that "Given the low wages paid to workers in service and clerical occupations, as well as students' perennial need for money, it is not surprising that most of the donors I interviewed found their interest in gamete donation sparked by donation program advertisements promising thousands of dollars" (Almeling 2008: 112). Eleven of the egg donors were employed in clerical, service work, or manual labor, four were unemployed while one was a salaried professional.

In the commercial egg and sperm market individuals select and purchase genetic material (egg and sperm) based on the physical and social characteristics of the egg and sperm donors. These characteristics include age, skin color, height, hair color, eye color, body shape, and perceived racial or ethnic origin. Consumers make choices about the desirability of specific egg and sperm donors who are socially classified on the basis of their presumed genetic heritage, skin color, body type, height, class background, age, educational achievement, and the physical appearance of children that they have produced. How do race, racism, social hierarchies, and religious beliefs shape choices regarding the selection of egg and sperm donors? National and colonial histories play a significant role in the criteria used by individuals and couples selecting egg donors. Social hierarchies travel across nation-states and become racialized in the consumption of commercial eggs. Racialized social hierarchies operate as decisions made about the desirability and attractiveness of egg donors.

Although neither eggs nor sperm possess skin color, yet their value is interpreted within hierarchies that privilege specific social characteristics. Sociologists have found that skin color (and particularly light or whiter skin) is a form of **symbolic capital** that has exchange value. In other words, light or White skin color can be converted into higher income, more education, marriage to higher-status men in both the Black and non-Black communities (Craig 2009; Glenn 2008; Thompson and Keith 2001). Sociologists have also demonstrated that lighter or White skin is more desirable and thus egg donors are classified in part by their skin tone, hair color, and eye color, and those individuals who possess lighter skin and more European or Asian features tend to be classified as "premium donors" and receive higher levels of compensation for their genetic material (Thompson 2005).

In an analysis of the use of skin tone as a criterion among individuals who use commercial egg donor databases, and in discussions with patients, donors, and clinic directors, Charis Thompson found that perceptions of "skin tone is not typically or only a perceptible physical property ... skin tone is inextricably tied up in transnational historical and geopolitical and religious bases of identity and relations of power" (2009: 147).

One example from Thompson's research involved a Japanese couple who traveled to the United States in order to purchase donated ova. In this case, the Japanese woman selected an Asian American egg donor based on her profile and her skin color, which was perceived as a good racial match. However, she changed her mind after learning that the parents of the egg donor were from Korea, a former colony of Japan. This knowledge about the ancestry of the donor altered her interpretation of the meaning of the skin tone. "The donor's light skin tone ceased to be attractive and desirable if it was not embedded in Japanese ancestry that gave the skin tone hierarchical meaning in the first place" (Thompson 2009: 143). Thus, the skin tone of Asian Americans of Korean ancestry was read by the Japanese as "not" an appropriate racial match due to their history of colonialism. Thompson argues that "Donors are chosen and compensated on the basis of desirable qualities, but many such qualities, especially ones like skin tone, are known to be highly unpredictably inherited" (Thompson 2009: 138).

Let us now shift the lens and view this process from the perspective of a Black woman who is seeking IVF due to her husband's sperm count. Black women and Jewish women often face obstacles that White Christian women don't face, because of the dearth of sperm that is considered "racially" and "religiously" a match. For example, if a Black Christian woman needs to purchase donor sperm in order to have a child her choices are restricted if she is forced to "racially match." She is often not given the same choices or degree of flexibility as "White" or Asian women. Seline Quiroga Szkupinski, a medical anthropologist, conducted research on Black, Latina, Asian, and Native American women seeking assistance with their fertility problems in the San Francisco Bay Area. Szkupinski identified practices that involved coercion and domination by White doctors while framing it in terms of individual choice. In her interviews with Black, Asian American, and Native Americans who were consumers of ART, she uncovered forms of policing by doctors that were recycled notions of racial purity, produced racial and ethnic boundaries, and enforced racial matching. For example, a Black woman she interviewed seeking IVF services was subjected to racial policing by the White doctors she consulted. The first doctor she consulted informed her that he didn't have any Black sperm donors so he couldn't offer her any sperm for IVF treatments. She was not allowed to purchase sperm provided by a non-Black donor. The White doctors appeared unable to recognize the great degree of skin color variation among Blacks and insisted that she must take the sperm from any Black donor regardless of whether they actually matched her husband's skin tone. This same woman argued that due to the racial mixing in most Black families "I would take a fair-skinned donor over a dark-skinned Black male, but what I am getting from the medical side is that they don't feel that's appropriate." The White doctors insisted that if a single Black male donor was available then it would be "inappropriate" for her to use "White" semen in IVF treatments (Szkupinski 2007: 153).[1]

In Israel, individuals are matched by religion and citizenship so only Israeli Jews can serve as sperm donors and/or surrogates for other Israeli Jewish couples. Research in Israel has also revealed that color hierarchies and national ideals become racialized via the practice of selecting and purchasing sperm from donors with idealized features. Michal Nahman conducted research on transnational ovum donation in two Israeli IVF clinics and a clinic in Romania that provided donor eggs for Jewish Israeli women (2005). In her analysis of the desired physical traits such as hair color, eye color, skin color, and height combined with interviews with women seeking to purchase "eggs" Nahman identified the ways that consumer choice is "linked to particular ideologies of race and racism" (2005: 210). Nahman argues that "In their consumption choices they utilized "Western forms of racial thinking" and thus reproduced European Christian ideals of beauty." According to Nahman a "technology of racism" operates in the physical traits that are idealized by the Jewish Israeli women who participated in this study. This technology of racism "extracts recipients' ideas about what is acceptable and not acceptable in the Jewish Israeli body" (Nahman 2005: 210). Her research participants preferred "light" or "White" skin. These same Jewish Israeli women rejected features that were perceived as "too Jewish," such as big noses and dark skin, and other features associated with Arabs and "Ethiopian Jews." Nahman argues that "many of my research participants expressed their wish not to have 'Black' babies" (Nahman 2005: 204).[2]

---

1 See Ratcliff (1989).

2 It is important to note that these ideals are not restricted to Israel but these ideals travel across national contexts. They can also be found in India and the United States. There is a sparse body of empirical literature specifically on this topic but the research that has been done suggests that White skin is privileged over other colors even in countries such as India where the majority of the population is brown (Thompson 2009).

Marcia Inhorn, a distinguished anthropologist who has conducted rigorous research on the infertility industry in Egypt, also found colorism and racism operating among Egyptian consumers of genetic materials. She notes that,

> Although Egypt is officially a "color-blind" society, with no explicit concept of "race" or racially based "minorities," veiled and not so veiled racism, especially towards individuals with dark skin and African features, is prevalent among Egyptians. Several elite women in my study made openly racist remarks to me during interviews, two of them using the English term "nigger." And such comments particularly surfaced around issues of [sperm] donation, as women described the racial "surprise" that might be in store for unwitting parents.

(Inhorn 2003: 113)

## DISCUSSION QUESTIONS

1. If you were considering hiring a gestational surrogate, how important would her race, education, skin color, and class be if she has no genetic relationship to the child for whom you are the intended parent?
2. Should the purchase price of genetic material (eggs and sperm) be regulated by the federal government? Do you think there should be limits on how much sperm or how many eggs can be donated by one individual?
3. How does the sale and consumption of genetic material differ from other forms of consumption? What ethical concerns do you have about this industry?
4. Do you think that children conceived with donated sperm that has been purchased have a right to know the identity of their genetic father when they reach 18 years of age? Why or why not?

# V: Religious Law and Regulatory Regimes

## Egypt and Israel

~~~~~~~~

What role does religion play in the infertility and assisted reproduction technology market in Egypt and Israel, two countries in the Middle East? How does religion and the state structure the IVF decisions for Egyptian and Israeli women? A comparative analysis of Egypt where gestational surrogacy is banned and Israel where it is state funded and completely regulated will shed light on this question.

The first Egyptian IVF center opened in 1986 in a wealthy suburb of Cairo. In 1987 Heba Mohammed, the first Egyptian test-tube baby, was born. In 1991, Shatby Hospital opened its first public IVF center and ten months later its first test-tube baby was born. However, despite the promise to provide state-subsidized fertility services to the poor, there is a low volume and most doctors have established private practices where they service the Egyptian elite while leaving the poor with no services. In Egypt, like the United States, there is a system of stratified reproduction. Only the most elite Egyptians, the top 1 percent of wage earners, can afford ART while the upper middle classes may be able to afford limited in vitro fertilization trials. The elite also have the resources to maintain their privacy so that they can hide their use of these services, which are stigmatized.

How do Egyptians find the money to pay for in vitro fertilization, which is very expensive in the wage structure of even educated middle class professionals? According to Inhorn, they utilize four strategies: 1) savings, 2) the sale of jewelry, 3) borrowing from family members, and 4) labor migration. Inhorn interviewed upper middle class Egyptians who were struggling to raise the money for IVF treatments. A significant segment of the middle class Egyptians who are able to afford IVF can do so because of labor migration. This is another difference between the United States and Egypt.

> The importance of labor migration to many IVF-seeking couples in this study cannot be underestimated, and it is one of the local features of test-tube baby making in Egypt that makes it very different from the West. For example, one Egyptian couple whom I interviewed together described how repeated, annual attempts to

make a test-tube baby would have never occurred without fourteen years of labor migration to Qatar, where he worked as an accountant and she as a nursery school teacher. Returning home on an annual, two-month vacation to Egypt, they finally succeeded with a twin pregnancy on their third trial of ICSI—a pregnancy that would have never occurred without Qatari money.

(Inhorn 2003: 43)

ICSI, intracytoplasmic sperm injection, is an IVF procedure used to treat male infertility in which a single sperm is injected directly into an egg. This couple spent $7,059, which is an exorbitant amount of money for middle class Egyptians and money that no one could obtain without becoming **wage exiles**.

In Egypt, in contrast to the United States, Israel and much of Europe, third party donation of eggs, sperm or embryos is religiously prohibited. **Procreative substances** (egg, sperm, and embryos) can only be combined if they belong to a married couple. These are viewed as moral imperatives and as necessary to preserve the marital bond and prevent genealogical "disruption" by introducing the sperm of another man into the womb of a married woman. This is done to:

- Preserve lineage (avoid confusion on issues of descent, inheritance, and kinship).
- Prevent future incestuous marriage of half-siblings fathered by same donor.
- Avoid reproduction outside of marriage, which is defined as adultery.
- Avoid third party donation, which is perceived as a threat to the marital bond.

Marcia Inhorn found that according to Islamic religious law,

Although third party donation does not involve the sexual "body contact" of adulterous relations, nor presumably the desire to engage in extramarital affairs, it is nonetheless considered by Islamic religious scholars to be a form of adultery, by virtue of introducing a third party into the sacred dyad of husband and wife.

(Inhorn 2003: 106–07)

Although Egypt, like Israel, is family-oriented and child-centered, it does not have a pronatalist state-funded system of reproductive health care. In contrast to Israel, a nation that has a more Western orientation than other nations in the Middle East, the Egyptian government does not provide subsidies for IVF. So Egypt is more comparable to the United States in terms of class disparities in relation to access to ART. Only the wealthy have access to IVF treatments in Egypt. And like those Americans who live in states where commercial surrogacy is prohibited, Egyptians have to travel to other countries in order to have access to some services, such as gestational surrogates.

Inhorn notes that,

[T]he mostly private nature of IVF services in Egypt has quickly engendered a three-tiered, class-based system of IVF accessibility, in which only the country's wealthy (as well as affluent Arabs from neighboring petro-rich nations) have unfettered access to the new assisted reproductive technologies now available. For middle-class and lower-class infertile Egyptians, having enough money to afford IVF or ICSI treatment is perhaps the fundamental arena of constraint limiting their ability to utilize these technologies—despite, in many cases, their ardent desire to do so.

(Inhorn 2003: 37)

Another difference between Egyptian Muslims and Christian views is that Muslims do not consider the destruction or "disposal" of unused embryos to be murder. Embryo cryopreservation was not available at the IVF centers where Inhorn conducted her research. "In short, in Egypt, the Islamic view on embryo disposal does not coincide with the Roman Catholic view that life begins at the moment of conception; thus, in the Muslim world, embryo disposal is not considered murder" (Inhorn 2003: 112).

Inhorn continues, "In making these local–global comparison, Egyptians, both Muslim and Coptic Christian, perceive themselves as morally superior to the Christian West, where in their opinion, 'the complete freedom' of medically assisted conception has created 'many problems'" (Inhorn 2003: 111). One of these problems is that according to this view, Americans treat the purchase of genetic material and the selection of sperm as if they are in a supermarket, which the Egyptians interviewed by Inhorn considered appalling.

Gestational surrogacy is *not* practiced in Egypt. From the perspective of Egyptians, both Muslim and Coptic Christians, the Christian West has lost its "moral compass" in a context in which there exists "complete freedom," and it has created a range of ethical problems. Egyptians interpret "rent-a-womb" arrangements as an exploitative international trade in adoptive babies, and assisting postmenopausal women to carry their own grandchildren as shocking and morally unacceptable. These "solutions" are seen as morally unacceptable among people who share the same problem of infertility. They disapprove of Western "banks of sperm" coded by race and color.

Cultural beliefs about social parenthood and particularly the prohibitions against adoption are inextricably linked to Islamic law and moral views of the use of sperm and ova from individuals who are not married (Inhorn 2003: 109). In the next section we will consider the role of religious law in Israel, which has taken a radically different approach from Egypt to commercial surrogacy.

## Israel: Rabbinic Law and State-Regulated Reproductive Technologies

Israel is the only country in the world that offers a program of government-subsidized new reproductive technologies to its citizens. Israel has been described as a nation that "has the most generous funding of IVF in the world" (Nahman 2005). All Israeli citizens, regardless of income, religion, or marital status are entitled to unlimited rounds of IVF treatment free of charge, up to the birth of two children (Inhorn 2003: 37).

In Israel, rabbinic law, or Jewish law, has been reconciled with new assisted reproductive technologies so that children born using these technologies can still be authorized as Jewish. Susan Kahn conducted an ethnographic study of the benefits that have accrued to Israeli Jewish women attempting to pursue motherhood as unmarried lesbians or heterosexuals in a pronatalist state that supports access to assisted reproductive technologies as a right of citizenship. She shows how unmarried Jewish lesbians have been able to access assisted reproductive technologies in a state that has given control over marriage and the family to religious authorities.

Kahn, an anthropologist, studied the ways that these technologies were conceptualized and reconciled with Halaka, Jewish law, and the flexibility of the Jewish kinship system. Kahn notes that, "By giving religious authorities jurisdiction over marriage and divorce in Israel, the secular government of a liberal, democratic, nation-state established a fundamental dependence upon Jewish religious law" (2000: 73). This is relevant because in Israel Jews can only marry other Jews—that is, individuals who are recognized by a rabbinical court as Jewish. This is a form of social exclusion and a restriction that bears directly upon the status of children conceived with the use of artificial insemination, embryo transfer, and other reproductive technologies. If an individual is conceived in a way that is not approved by rabbinical courts or defined as "illicit," which would include adulterous, incestuous unions, then they are considered mamzers, a social stigma. Mamzers are not marriageable for ten generations.

> These technologies have the potential to challenge entrenched notions and the appropriate relationship between marriage and its role in reproduction. The Israeli case is remarkable in that efforts to legislate for the appropriate uses of these technologies have revealed unusual points of consensus between traditional Jewish law and progressive secular law. Most strikingly, both legal systems grant varying measures of reproductive agency to unmarried women … they force potentially subversive underpinnings of Jewish kinship reckoning to become explicit. We have seen how these dynamics have unleashed the reproductive agency of unmarried women … Orthodox rabbi maybe object to the deliberate insemination of unmarried women out of concern for the protection of the traditional nuclear family, but their arguments have no legal foundation in religious law.
>
> (Kahn 2000: 84–85)

In 1994 the **Aloni Commission Report** was published in Israel. This government-sponsored report had been commissioned by the Ministry of Justice to examine the ethical, legal, social, and religious issues surrounding surrogacy. The Aloni report established a national level committee that would supervise and regulate surrogacy contracts a priori. This report, like the Warnock Report in England and the Glover Report for the European Commission, examined the legal, social, ethical, and religious issues relating to the uses of assistive reproductive technologies. Unlike the Warnock Report in England, a major goal of this report was to bring the legislation of reproductive technologies into alignment with Jewish and Israeli law.

This report established the following rights for *unmarried* women:

1. Right to privacy.
2. Every Israeli is granted the right to receive state-subsidized fertility treatments.
3. Marital status cannot be used to deny access to fertility treatments.

The Aloni Commission Report established several fundamental rights for Israelis that bear directly upon the ability of *unmarried* Jewish women to have children who are recognized by rabbinical courts as "Jewish." These two clear principles are relevant for all Jewish Israeli women. First, "the right to privacy." This right to reproductive agency is thus legally defined as a basic human right in a progressive secular society. This is a right that most poor women in the United States still don't possess since they may not have the financial resources to access contraception, abortion, or fertility treatments. Second, this report guarantees access for everyone to fertility. The report reads, the "right to receive fertility treatment should be granted to every person" (Kahn 2000: 77). Thus, in contrast to the United States and much of Europe, an individual's lack of wealth and social class does not exclude them from access to ART. In the United States it has primarily been the upper middle classes and the wealthy who can afford to purchase the medical, legal, and travel expenses related to surrogacy. And the right to privacy remains at risk for women seeking abortion as a form of reproductive control.

Two dissenting opinions attached to this report expressed concern regarding the creation of "socially defective" offspring. One concern raised by Rabbi Halperin, who wrote one of the dissenting opinions for the Aloni Commission, is that children produced using anonymous Jewish sperm would unwittingly marry one of their half-siblings in the future. This is a serious concern that could require future DNA testing of children conceived via anonymous sperm donation prior to marriage. At this time ART is regulated via secondary legislation rather than formal legislation.

Although the vast majority of Jews in Israel are secular, and according to Kahn, "those who seek fertility treatments do not consult rabbis for guidance," rabbinic authority remains important because the Jewishness of children born using assisted conception must meet the approval of a rabbinical court in cases of dispute. Moreover, since religious courts hold this authority and orthodox Jews may use these technologies in consultation with their rabbis, "orthodox Jews have constructed elaborate, independent frameworks for the administration of these technologies, frameworks that depend on close cooperation between fertility specialists, orthodox rabbis, and infertile orthodox patients" (Kahn 2000: 89).

The surrogacy industry in Israel is organized by a system of religious and ethnic segregation. When orthodox couples consult rabbinic counselors at orthodox-run fertility clinics they are "ethnically" matched to an Ashkenazi or Sephardic rabbi based upon whether they are Sephardic or Ashkenazi. Couples with the same fertility problems may receive permission for different treatment options due to the unique circumstances of their case including their age, health issues, etc. Although the vast majority of Jews are secular in Israel, for Orthodox religiously observant Jews, the potential social stigma that could attach to a child conceived via ART without rabbinic approval is profound. Rabbinic approval is required before the state committee will approve of the fertility treatments and this is required to guarantee that any resultant children are recognized as "Jewish" and thus eligible for marriage in their community. The Israeli government provides unmarried women with the same rights of access to ART as married women. In Kahn's analysis this right to reproduce with state support "lays the legal framework for a profound social reimagination of the nuclear family as a prerequisite for reproduction." Kahn continues:

> If the state explicitly constructs reproduction as an individual right, then the nuclear family becomes simply one structural option for reproduction among many. And as soon as the nuclear family ceases to be legally privileged as the locus for reproduction the potential exists that it will cease to be socially privileged in other ways.

(Kahn 2000: 83)

The children of unmarried Jewish women are not considered "illegitimate" and thus children conceived via ART by unmarried women retain their Jewishness, according to rabbinical law. As a consequence, unmarried Jewish Israeli women have protected legal rights under rabbinical law that they do not possess in the United States. Moreover, their status as single mothers is not necessarily viewed as a "spoiled identity" since their children are recognized as Jewish and thus marriageable in Israel.

## The Surrogate Motherhood Agreements Law

In 1996 Israel passed **The Surrogate Motherhood Agreements Law** and became the first nation in the world to facilitate state-financed commercial surrogacy agreements. The first birth from a surrogacy contract took place in February 1998. The Surrogate Agreements Law does not give any legal status to the birth mother upon the child's birth. The Law allows only for gestational surrogacy agreements, thereby forbidding traditional surrogacy. The sperm must be from the "intended" father.

When the Israeli government legalized gestational surrogacy in March 1996, it became the first country in the world to implement a regulatory regime in which each and every surrogacy contract must be approved by the state. Israel has more commercial surrogacy centers per capita than any other country.

## Access to ART by Unmarried Women: Legal Challenges by Israeli Lesbians

In a study of assisted conception in Israel, the U.S. anthropologist Susan Martha Kahn notes that,

> The ministry of health regulations differ from the Aloni Commission's recommendation in that they *attach intrusive restrictions to single women's right of access to these technologies.* Thus although the state legitimized and guaranteed that single women will not be denied right of access to reproductive technology simply because they are unmarried, the state retained for itself a form of control over single women's reproductive agency.

> (emphasis added; Kahn 2000: 80)

In a 1996 legal case brought before the Israeli High Court by the Association for Civil Rights in Israel on behalf of a lesbian plaintiff, restrictions placed on unmarried women but not on married women were challenged. In this case an unmarried lesbian mother of two children was asked to undergo a psychiatric evaluation in addition to social worker evaluation in order to get pre-approval for state-funded sperm donation. Dr. Tal Yarus-Haka challenged this rule, stating that since it was only required of unmarried women this constituted a violation of her right to procreate and discriminated against her on the basis of her marital status and thus violated her civil rights. The Israeli Supreme Court ruled on behalf of this lesbian mother (Kahn 2000: 81–82).

Based upon her analysis of this legal case and another involving unmarried women who had successfully challenged restrictions on their access to sperm donation, Kahn concludes that

> The Israeli case is remarkable in that efforts to legislate for the appropriate uses of these technologies have *revealed unusual points of consensus between traditional Jewish law and progressive secular law.* Most strikingly, both legal systems grant varying measures of reproductive agency to unmarried women ... The policing of the family is thus left to the conceptual imagination of a diverse array of social actors, from orthodox rabbis to secular legislators to unmarried women themselves.

> (emphasis added; Kahn 2000: 85)

In the first study of gestational surrogacy in Israel, Teman argues that

> The cultural anxieties provoked by surrogacy in relation to the family are further amplified by the anxieties surrogacy raises over loss of maternal wholeness, as the perceived unity of motherhood is deconstructed in surrogacy and the parts distributed among at least three potential mothers: genetic, gestational, and social. Giving birth to a child for the purpose of relinquishment also defies mainstream assumptions that identify pregnancy with the birth mother's commitment to the project of subsequent lifelong mothering and threaten dominant ideologies in many cultures that assume an indissoluble mother-child bond.

(Teman 2010: 7)

The issue of religion obviously plays a central role in conferring Jewishness upon the child. Israeli surrogates are more likely to be unmarried and to be employed. They may be steadily employed or temporarily employed. They are slightly older than U.S. surrogates and ethnically matched. They tend to share the same ethnicity, meaning if they are Arab or Sephardic Jew then they would serve as a surrogate for another Arab or Sephardic Jew. The class gap is typically smaller between surrogates and the "intended" mother in comparison to the United States.

## DISCUSSION QUESTIONS

1. What role, if any, should religious bodies play in the regulation of assisted reproductive technologies in the United States? Do you think we should follow Israel as a model?
2. What advantages do you see to having the federal government set up a regulatory commission to pre-approve all surrogacy contracts in advance?
3. Do you think income should be a barrier to forming a family? If you answer is no, should poor married people have the same access to assisted reproductive technologies as upper middle class married heterosexual couples?
4. If you think the government should support childless couples in accessing ART, should the government also restore funding for abortions for women who are already parents and don't have the resources to support more children?

# VI:  India

## A View from the Global South

⤜⋆⤛

On July 25, 2009 Manji Yamada, a little girl who became known as "Baby M," was born in Anand. Her birth generated a constitutional crisis in Indian courts due to the fact that her contractual parents had divorced before her birth. She became a **surrogate orphan** with no legal parents and no citizenship status. The baby's parents, Ikufumi Yamada, 45, and his wife Yuki Yamada, entered into a surrogacy agreement and hired the services of a surrogate while married. Before the birth they separated and then divorced. Yuki Yamada is not genetically related to the child, because an Indian woman donated the ovum, while Ikufumi Yamada provided the sperm. Indian law does not permit an unmarried man to adopt a female infant. This created a legal situation in which Baby M had no legal mother and thus her citizenship was in dispute. On August 20, the Supreme Court of India granted the custody of Baby M to Emiko Yamada, her 74-year-old grandmother.

Within the past three years Anand, a city in the State of Gujarat in western India, has emerged as a transnational hub for surrogacy. Although California remains the global destination of choice for reproductive tourists seeking gestational surrogates, Anand has quickly developed an international profile as a destination where gestational surrogates can be hired at cheaper prices compared to the U.S. by consumers from Canada, Israel, Japan, India, Germany, and the Middle East as well as the United States and other parts if Europe. Describing the Indian surrogacy market, Amrita Pande, an Indian-American sociologist fluent in Hindi and Gujarati, writes "The Indian structure is closest to the liberal market model of surrogacy in California where surrogacy births are primarily managed by private, commercial agencies that screen, match, and regulate agreements according to their own criteria and without state interference" (2009a: 382).

The 2010 documentary, *Google Baby*, produced by Israeli Zippi Brand Frank, follows Doron, a gay Israeli entrepreneur who provides services to gay men in Israel who want to form a family. His customers purchase the eggs and sperm online and the babies are delivered in India. The viewer sees Israeli men viewing egg donor profiles of White U.S. women and purchasing ova to be gestated in the wombs of Indian surrogates in the Akanksha Clinic in Anand. The women who work as reproductive laborers in the Akanksha Clinic in India spend their entire pregnancies in guarded and cloistered residential facilities.

How does the experience of gestational surrogates in India differ from those of the Israeli and American surrogates? Amrita Pande conducted field research in Anand between 2006 and 2008. Pande interviewed 42 gestational surrogates, their husbands, in-laws, and two surrogacy brokers in a groundbreaking study. The women interviewed by Pande were much poorer than their Israeli and American counterparts. Like U.S. and Israeli gestational surrogates, they had all given birth and were the mothers of at least one child. In contrast, however, they were all married and they had much less education, ranging from illiterate to high school education. Most were also impoverished. So rather than being working class or lower middle class, they were living at the poverty line as defined by the Indian government. Pande describes their income thus, "For most of the surrogates' families, the money earned through surrogacy was equivalent to five years of total family income" (Pande 2010: 974).

We learn several things from Pande's study. First, in contrast to the U.S., Israel, and Europe, surrogacy appears to be a very stigmatized occupation in India. According to Pande this motivates Indian surrogates to reside in dormitories in seclusion during their contract pregnancies:

> In India, however, surrogates face a high amount of stigma. As a consequence, almost all the surrogates in this study except one decided to keep their surrogacy a secret from their communities, villages, and, very often, from their parents. They usually hid in the clinic or took temporary accommodation away from their communities during the last months of pregnancy.
>
> (2009b: 154)

Second, Pande introduces the concept of **sexualized care work** "to describe a new type of reproductive labor—commercial surrogacy—that is similar to existing forms of care work but is stigmatized in the public imagination, among other reasons, because of its parallel with sex work" (Pande 2010: 142). Pande found that the Indian surrogates she interviewed emphasized their maternal connection to the babies they gestated. Rather than emphasizing the genetic tie that the child had to the intended mother, they argued that they had a maternal bond with the child because they *shared bodily substances (blood/breast milk)* and had labored to give birth to these babies. In contrast to enslaved U.S. Black women who served as wet nurses during slavery, as employed workers these women received wages for their labor, yet Pande argues that they rejected this status as a contract laborer. Pande argues that they employed discourses that minimized their role (and identity) as contract workers. Pande characterizes this as a "disruption" to gender hierarchies that privilege the genetic father's sperm and the genetic mother. They insist upon their shared blood during pregnancy, their labor and breastfeeding as the basis for their maternal connection with the children.

In contrast to the Israeli surrogates interviewed by Teman, they redefine kinship to emphasize the non-procreative basis (Pande 2009a).

Pande's most significant finding and what distinguishes Indian surrogates from their Israeli counterparts is the issue of stigma. The Indian surrogates employed a moral discourse to manage this. According to Pande, "the surrogates affirmed their dignity and sense of self-worth and reduced the stigma attached to surrogacy" by reinforcing gender inequalities that denied that they were contract laborers who earned a wage (Pande 2010). Pande offers insights into why Indian surrogates don't develop a worker's identity as commercial surrogates.

If we compare Indian surrogates to the Israeli surrogates interviewed by Teman, the issue of stigma did not seem to be significant in Israel. In Israel, where surrogacy is state-regulated and motherhood exalted, gestational surrogacy is not a stigmatized occupation. The cult of motherhood in Israel and the pronatalist state imperatives has generated a very different set of issues for Israeli surrogates.

Helena Ragoné (1994) published the first and only book-length study of gestational surrogates in the United States. The limited studies that we have of U.S. surrogates suggest that egg donors may be more stigmatized than gestational surrogates by family members. In other words, selling one's genetic material may be perceived as different from performing "labor" for an infertile couple in need. There is some anecdotal evidence from journalistic reports that some U.S. Black women must manage the stigma that their Black relatives attach to surrogacy, particularly when they are carrying a child for White Europeans or European-Americans. Given the long history of slavery and exploitation of Black women's reproductive labor by White Americans, this occupation may not be viewed as acceptable within the Black community, but to date there are no studies examining this issue from the perspective of U.S. Black surrogates. Pande's findings call attention to the dearth of ethnographic studies of gestational surrogacy that illuminate the experiences of Black, Mexican-American, Puerto Rican, Latina, and other women who socially classified as members of racial or ethnic minorities who are oppressed in the U.S.

## DISCUSSION QUESTIONS

1. Identify and describe one significant difference between the gestational surrogacy markets in India and Israel. If you were seeking employment as a gestational surrogate where would you want to work India, Israel, or the U.S.? Why?

2. Pande found that Indian surrogates emphasized their maternal bond with the "surrogate" child they were paid to bear. Why do you think they minimized their status as paid reproductive laborers?

# VII:   Reproductive Justice and Reproductive Liberty

The global market in gestational surrogacy has generated a new set of ethical dilemmas and sociological questions regarding the responsibility of the state, the commercial agencies that broker these contracts, contracting parents and the rights of gestational surrogates. Individuals who have the financial resources are able to exercise their reproductive agency in ways that those lacking economic and political power and forms of social capital are not. Thus, access to reproductive technologies remains restricted, in most cases, to the most powerful. There are, of course, exceptions, as we saw in the case of Israel, which has established a state-controlled regulatory body that provides more democratic access in comparison to the free-market system in the United States, which renders forming a family using assisted reproductive technologies a privilege rather than a procreative right to which everyone is entitled.

Should access to assisted reproductive technologies be a right? Should it be included in basic health care that is state funded? Should wealthy people of the upper middle classes have privileged access to the bodies of less privileged women? How should this industry be regulated? Is an international body to regulate it an invasion of the privacy of citizens of nation-states? Commercial surrogacy continues to be controversial and poses a range of ethical questions even as the industry expands. At the time of writing Sweden is currently debating legalizing commercial surrogacy.

Pande argues that "These (Eurocentric) portrayals of surrogacy cannot incorporate the reality of a developing country setting—where commercial surrogacy has become a survival strategy and a temporary occupation for some poor women" (2009b: 144). While Pande is correct that there is a need to understand this industy from the perspective of India, I disagree that ethics are not relevant here and that considering them is Eurocentric. Pande does not comment on the parallels between poor Indian women and poor women of color in the United States who are reproductive laborers in this industry.

If we consider the issue of surrogacy from the perspective of poor men and women who are infertile or anyone who does not possess the economic resources to purchase ART services or to travel to another region or nation-state to purchase these services at a lower cost, we see that ART remains restricted to a global elite. It is a commodity that is out of reach of a vast majority of people who have fertility problems as well as single gay men or same sex male couples who wish to form a family to which they have a genetic tie.

In her analysis of the U.S. debate over whether to legalize or ban commercial surrogacy, Susan Markens notes that this debate is best understood as a larger debate about the meaning of motherhood, parenting, and the family. She notes that:

> [T]he way the social problem of surrogate parenting was framed also reveals important *similarities* in both sides' views about families and in the dominant cultural beliefs they chose to use when advocating for their respective positions. In particular, both surrogacy supporters and opponents drew on their dominant ideology of a public/private divide, in which the family was understood to occupy the private realm. As a result, both frames reinforced the idea that relationships pursued and formed in families should not be interfered with by the outside world. At the same time, in evoking privacy rights, both sides often ignored how such individually based rights historically have upheld racial and class privilege
>
> (Markens 2007: 91)

What is relevant here is that if we compare this to the Israeli case, we see that the right to privacy was also used to support the rights of women to have access to ART *and* to have it state funded. The issue of privacy is often viewed as American; however, as Markens correctly notes, the right to privacy is typically used to reinforce and restore the privileges of the racially dominant groups to reproduce while restricting or denying the poor and ethnic minorities those same rights.

## Towards a Reproductive Rights Model

Who has the right to reproduce? Should only those who have the financial resources to pay for assisted reproduction be able to reproduce? Or should we assist all citizens of childbearing age to form families? Is access to assisted reproductive technologies a right and a privilege or are they a resource that should be evenly distributed? We have learned that in Israel, a pronatalist state that strictly controls marriage, the government provides subsidies to support in vitro fertilization and supports gestational surrogacy for Israeli citizens regardless of their income, marital status, or sexual orientation. From the perspective of Israeli Jewish citizens this is a more economically democratic approach. In contrast, we have seen that the U.S. fertility industry is structured by racial and class inequality and that is a stratified system that denies access to large segments of the population that do not possess the financial resources to purchase these services. Assisted reproductive technologies are typically only available to the economically privileged who in most cases are also the racially dominant groups in the United States.

*But to gladly take the IVF subsidies?*

Feminists, philosophers, and critical legal scholars have debated the meaning of liberty and the role of procreation in liberty. Is procreation a constitutional right? If one is poor and does not have the resources to pay for reproductive health care, including access to abortion or fertility services, one is not able to exercise procreative agency. Furthermore, in the case of enslaved women in the past, their children did not belong to them and thus, they did not exercise or what Dorothy Roberts, a legal scholar and critical race theorist, calls "reproductive liberty." In the United States reproductive liberty has been reserved for the wealthy and historically for White affluent women in particular.

In *Killing the Black Body: Race, Reproduction and the Meaning of Liberty*, Dorothy Roberts argues for a rethinking of the meaning of liberty. According to Roberts, the experience of Black women and men has been one in which they have been denied reproductive control over their bodies and reproductive liberty. She argues that **structural racism** should be taken into account in discussion of reproduction. In her words, "white racism has perverted dominant notions of reproductive freedom, the quest to secure Black women's reproductive autonomy can transform the meaning of liberty for everyone" (Roberts 1998: 7).

Roberts advocates for the following:

*what about the ability to support children?*

- State support for the procreative decisions of poor women that include both funding to terminate pregnancies and funding for ART and IVF.
- Removal of economic barriers to in vitro fertilization which is costly and in the United States only available to the most economically and racially privileged members of society.
- Provide government subsidies to poor families so that they can afford IVF.

Robertson (1994), a philosopher, sees "**procreative liberties**" as negative rights, that is the right "against state interference" in procreative decisions, whether the decision is to have children or to avoid having them. It is a primary liberty.

In a comparative analysis of Egypt and the United States, we find that Egypt, a resource-poor nation, shares several striking similarities with the U.S. in terms of restricted access to assisted reproductive technologies. Marcia Inhorn provides an instructive comparative case that demonstrates how wealth and poverty structure the reproductive choices of non-elites. Elite Egyptians like their U.S. counterparts are able to purchase reproductive services, travel to other countries to purchase services (Americans can travel to other states or nations if their state bans commercial surrogacy), and maintain their privacy while these same services are unavailable to poorer Egyptians.

## DISCUSSION QUESTIONS

1. Should the U.S. government provide access to ART and subsidies to assist poor women to form a family, regardless of their marital status or sexual orientation, as they do in Israel?
2. Do you consider assisted reproductive technologies a procreative right or a privilege?

# Bibliography

Ali, Lorraine, and Raina Kelley. 2008. "The Curious Lives of Surrogates." Cover story for *Newsweek* (April 7): 45–51.

Allen, Anita. 1991. "The Black Surrogate Mother." *Harvard Blackletter Journal 8*: 17–31.

Almeling, Rene. 2008. "Selling Genes, Selling Gender: Egg Donation, Sperm Donation, and the Medical Market in Genetic Material," unpublished Ph.D. dissertation, University of California at Los Angeles (UCLA).

*American Heritage Dictionary of the English Language,* 3rd edition. 1996 (1992). Boston/New York: Houghton Mifflin Company.

Andrews, Lori. 1989. *Between Strangers: Surrogate Mothers, Expectant Fathers, and Brave New Babies.* New York: Harper & Row.

Baker, Brenda. 1996. "A Case for Permitting Altruistic Surrogacy." *Hypatia: A Journal of Feminist Philosophy 11*(2): 34–48.

Bellafante, Gina. 2005. "Surrogate Mothers' New Niche: Bearing Babies for Gay Couples." *The New York Times* (May 25).

Bosely, Sarah. 2004. "Donor Children Will Have Right to Know." *Guardian* (January 22). Available online (www.guardian.co.uk).

Carney, Scott. 2010. "Cash on Delivery." *Mother Jones* (March/April): 69–73.

Center for Disease Control. 2006. *Assisted Reproductive Technology Success Rates.* Atlanta, GA: US Department of Health and Human Services, Center for Disease Control and Prevention. Available online (www.cdc.gov/art/ART2006/PDF/2006ART.pdf).

Chelser, Phyliss. 1988. *Sacred Bond.* New York: Times Books.

Colen, Shellee. 1995. "Like a Mother to Them: Stratified Reproduction and West Indian Childcare Workers and Employers in New York." Pp. 78–102 in *Conceiving the New World Order: The Global Politics of Reproduction,* eds. Faye D. Ginsburg and Rayna Rapp. Berkeley and Los Angeles: University of Chicago Press.

Cook, Rachel, Shelley Day Sclater, with Felicity Kaganas, eds. 2003. *Surrogate Motherhood: International Perspectives.* Portland, OR: Hart Publishing.

Corea, Gena. 1985. *The Mother Machine: Reproductive Technologies from Artificial Insemination to Artificial Wombs.* New York: Harper & Row.

Craig, Maxine Leeds. 2009. "The Color of an Ideal Negro Beauty Queen: Miss Bronze 1961–1968." Pp. 81–94 in *Shades of Difference: Why Skin Color Matters,* ed. Evelyn Nakano Glenn. Stanford: Stanford University Press.

*Economic Times*. 2007. "Giving Birth Becomes the Latest Job Outsourced to India as Commercial Surrogacy Takes off." *Economic Times* (December 30).

Field, Martha A. 1990. *Surrogate Motherhood*. Cambridge, MA: Harvard University Press.

Franklin, Sarah. 1997. *Embodied Progress: A Cultural Account of Assisted Conception*. London: Routledge.

Gentleman, Amelia. 2008. "India Nurtures Business of Surrogate Motherhood." *The New York Times* (March 10).

Ginsburg, Faye, and Rayna Rapp, eds. 1995. *Conceiving the New World Order: The Global Politics of Reproduction*. Berkeley/Los Angeles/London: University of California Press.

Glenn, Evelyn Nakano. 1992. "From Servitude to Service Work: Historical Continuities in the Division of Labor." *Signs: Journal of Women in Culture and Society* 18(1): 1–43.

———. 2008. "Yearning for Lightness: Transnational Circuits in the Marketing and Consumption of Skin Lighteners." *Gender and Society* 22(3) (June): 281–302.

Goslinga-Roy, Gillian. 2000. "Body Boundaries, Fiction of the Female Self: An Ethnography of Power, Feminism and the Reproductive Technologies." *Feminist Studies* 26(1) (Spring): 113–40.

Grayson, Deborah. 1998. "'Mediating Intimacy: Black Surrogate Mothers and the Law." *Critical Inquiry* 24 (Winter): 540.

Hartouni, Valerie. 1994. "Breached Birth: Reflections on Race, Gender and Reproductive Discourse in the 1980s." *Configurations* 2(1): 73–88.

Hendricks, Jennifer. S. 2007. "Essentially a Mother." *William and Mary Journal of Women and the Law 13*: 429–82.

Hochschild, Arlie Russell, with Anne Machung. 2003 (1989). *The Second Shift*. New York: Penguin Books.

Horsbourgh, Beverly. 1993. "Jewish Women, Black Women: Guarding against Oppression of Surrogacy." *Berkeley Women's Law Journal* 8(29): 29–62.

Inhorn, Marcia. 1995. *Infertility and Patriarchy: The Cultural Politics of Gender and Family Life in Egypt*. Philadelphia: University of Pennsylvania Press.

———. 2003. *Local Babies, Global Science: Gender, Religion and In Vitro Fertilization*. New York: Routledge.

Inhorn, Marcia, and Frank van Balen. 2002. *Infertility around the Globe: New Thinking on Childlessness, Gender and Reproductive Technologies*. Berkeley/Los Angeles: University of California Press.

Kahn, Susan Martha. 2000. *Reproducing Jews: A Cultural Account of Assisted Conception in Israel*. Durham and London: Duke University Press.

Kandel, R. F. 1994. "Which Came First? The Mother or the Egg? A Kinship Solution to Gestational Surrogacy." *Rutgers Law Review 47*: 165.

Krucoff, Carol. 1983. "The Surrogate Baby Boom." *Washington Post* (January 25): Section C: 5.

Kuczynski, Alex. 2008. "Her Body, My Baby: My Adventures with a Surrogate Mom." *The New York Times Magazine* (November 20): 42.

Laukfer-Ukeles, Pamela. 2002. "Gestation: Work for Hire or the Essence of Motherhood: A Comparative Legal Analysis." *Duke Journal of Gender, Law and Policy 9*: 91–134.

Liebler, Raizel. 2002. "Are you my Parent? Are you my Child?: The Role of Genetics and Race in Defining Relationships after Reproductive Technological Mistakes." *DePaul Journal Health Care and Law 15*: 25.

McKinley, Jesse. 1998. "The Egg Woman." *The New York Times* (May 17): Section 14: 1.

Markens, Susan. 2007. *Surrogate Motherhood and the Politics of Reproduction.* Berkeley/Los Angeles/London: University of California Press.

Marx, Karl. 1967. *Capital: A Critique of Political Economy.* New York: International Publishers.

May, Elaine Taylor. 1997. *Barren in the Promised Land: Childless Americans and the Pursuit of Happiness.* Cambridge, MA: Harvard University Press.

Morgan, Derek. 2003. "Enigma Variations: Surrogacy, Rights and Procreative Tourism." Pp. 75–92 in *Surrogated Motherhood: International Perspectives,* eds. Rachel Cook, Shelley Day Sclater, with Felicity Kaganas. Portland, Oregon: Hart Publishing.

Nahman, Michal. 2005. "Materializing Israeliness: Difference and Mixture in Transnational Ova Donation." *Science as Culture 15*(3): 199–213.

Oliver, Kelly. 1989. "Marxism and Surrogacy." *Hypatia 4*(3) (Fall): 95–115.

Overall, Christine. 1987. *Ethics and Human Reproduction: A Feminist Analysis.* Boston: Allen and Unwin.

Pande, Amrita. 2009a. "'It May be her Eggs but it's my Blood': Surrogates and Everyday Forms of Kinship in India." *Qualitative Sociology 32*(4): 379–404.

———. 2009b. "Not an Angel, Not a Whore: Surrogates as 'Dirty Workers' in India." *Indian Journal of Gender Studies 16*(2): 141–73.

———. 2010. "Commercial Surrogacy in India: Manufacturing a Perfect Mother-Worker." *Signs 35*(4) (Summer): 969–92.

Parrenas, Rhacel Salazar, and Boris, Eileen. 2010. *Intimate Labors: Cultures, Technologies and the Politics of Care.* Stanford: Stanford University Press.

Pelka, Suzanne. 2005. *Lesbian Couples Creating Families using In Vitro Fertilization to Co-Mother: A Cultural Study of Biological Ties.* Unpublished doctoral dissertation. University of Chicago.

Radin, M. J. 1996. *Contested Commodities: The Trouble with the Trade in Sex, Children, Bodily Parts and Other Things.* Cambridge, MA: Harvard University Press.

Ragoné, Helena. 1994. *Surrogate Motherhood: Conception in the Heart.* Boulder, CO: Westview Press.

———. 2000. "Of Likeness and Difference: How Race is being Transfigured by Gestational Surrogacy." Pp. 56–75 in *Ideologies and Technologies of Motherhood,* eds. Helena Ragoné and France Winddance Twine. New York: Routledge.

Ratcliff, Kathryn Strother, ed. 1989. *Healing Technology: Feminist Perspectives.* Ann Arbor: University of Michigan.

Roberts, Dorothy. 1995. "The Genetic Tie." *University of Chicago Law Review 62*: 209–73.

———. 1998. *Killing the Black Body: Race, Reproduction and the Meaning of Liberty.* New York: Vintage Books.

Robertson, J. A. 1994. *Children of Choice: Freedom and the New Reproductive Technologies.* Princeton, NJ: Princeton University Press.

Rosenblatt, Roger. 1987. "Baby M—Emotions for Sale." *Time* magazine (Monday, April 6).

Rotabi, Karen Smith. 2010. "Human Rights and the Business of Reproduction: Surrogacy Replacing International Adoption from Guatemala." Retrieved May 20, 2010 (www.rhrealitycheck.org/blog/).

Rousseau, Nicole. 2009. *Black Women's Burden: Commodifying Black Reproduction.* New York: Palgrave Macmillan.

Sanders, Cheryl J. 1992. "Surrogate Motherhood and Reproductive Technologies: An African American Perspective." *Creighton Law Review 25*: 1707–23.

Singer, P., and D. Wells. 1984. *The Reproduction Revolution: New Ways of Making Babies.* Oxford: Oxford University Press.

Smith, Nicole. 2010. "'Inside the Baby Farm: Childless Couples from around the World are Traveling to India to Have Babies by Surrogate Mothers." *The Sunday Times,* magazine section (London), national edition: 22, 23, 25, 27, and 29.

Solinger, Rickie. 2000. *Wake Up Little Susie: Race and Single Pregnancy Before Roe v. Wade.* New York/London: Routledge.

Spar, Deborah. 2006. *The Baby Business: How Money, Science and Politics Drive the Commerce of Conception.* Boston, MA: Harvard Business School Press.

Szkupinski, Seline Quiroga. 2007. "Blood is Thicker than Water: Policing Donor Insemination and the Reproduction of Whiteness." *Hypatia: A Journal of Feminist Philosophy 22*(2) (March): 143–57.

Teman, Ely. 2010. *Birthing the Mother: The Surrogate Body and the Pregnant Self.* Berkeley: University of California Press.

Thompson, Charis. 2005. *Making Parents: The Ontological Choreography of Reproductive Technologies.* Cambridge, MA: Massachusetts Institute of Technology.

———. 2009. "Skin Tone and the Persistence of Biological Race in Egg Donation for Assisted Reproduction." Pp. 131–47 in *Shades of Difference: Why Skin Color Matters,* ed. Evelyn Nakano Glenn. Stanford: Stanford University Press.

Thompson, Maxine S., and Keith, Verna. 2001. "The Blacker the Berry: Gender, Skin Tone, Self-Esteem ad Self-Efficacy." *Gender and Society 15*: 336–57.

Tran, Max. 2000. "Fertility Laws." *Guardian* (February 14). Available online (www.guardian.co.uk).

Wald, Jenny. 1997. "Outlaw Mothers." *Hastings Women's Law Journal 8*: 169.

Warner, Judith. 2008. "Outsourced Wombs." *The New York Times* (January 3).

Warnock, Mary. 1985. *A Question of Life: The Warnock Report on Human Fertilisation and Embryology.* Oxford: Basil Blackwell.

Weisberg, Kelly D. 2005. *The Birth of Surrogacy in Israel.* Gainseville, FL: University Press of Florida.

Weiss, M. 2002. *The Chosen Body: The Politics of the Body in Israeli Society.* Stanford: Stanford University Press.

Zelizer, Viviana. A. 1988. "Beyond the Polemics on the Market: Establishing a Theoretical and Empirical Agenda," *Sociological Forum 3* (Fall): 614–34.

# Glossary/Index

~~~~~~~~

**A**

**Aloni Commission Report:** in 1991 the Aloni Commission was established in Israel by the Ministers of Health and Justice. They were asked to study assisted reproductive technologies including in vitro fertilization and to propose legislation to regulate assisted reproductive technologies. In 1994 they submitted their report to the Ministers of Health and Justice. This report established a national committee to regulate state funded surrogacy contracts and unlimited IVF trials up to the birth of two children. 41

**assisted reproductive technologies (ART):** this term generally refers to asexual reproduction—achieving pregnancy and birth without sexual intercourse. The Center for Disease Control defines ART as "all fertility treatments in which both eggs and sperm are handled. In general ART procedures involve surgically removing eggs from a woman's ovaries, combining them with sperm in the laboratory, and returning them to the woman's body or donating them to another woman" (2006: 3). ART includes the following technologies: 1) intrauterine insemination, 2) donation of eggs, 3) donation of sperm), 4) in vitro fertilization and the transfer of the embryos, and 6) intracytoplasmic sperm injection. 2

**B**

*The Baby Business* 7
Baby M case, India 45
Baby M case, U.S. 4
    legacy of trial 5–7
biblical examples of surrogacy 13
birth certificates 11
    in Baby M case 5, 6
*Birthing a Mother* 26
Black women
    Caribbean child care workers in New York 3
    denied reproductive liberty 8, 13–14, 50
    racist experiences in seeking IVF services 34–35
    and stigma of surrogacy 47
    vulnerabilities as surrogates 14–15
    White surrogates advantaged over 16
bodily integrity, strategies for 27–28
**body map:** a conceptual tool employed by gestational surrogates to manage interpersonal boundaries between themselves and the couples for whom they are carrying pregnancies to term. It enables them to distinguish between parts of the body they wish to personalize and the parts that they wish to distance, both cognitively and emotionally. Elly Teman found that Israeli surrogates employ the body map as a tool during pregnancy to conduct "emotion work" that distances them from the fetuses. 27
*Brave New World* 1, 4
Brown, Louise 5

**C**

Carney, Scott 17
Center for Disease Control 11
children
    commodification of 8, 16
    legitimacy laws 42
class
    and access to ART 7–8, 10, 38–39, 41, 49
    and divisions in reproductive labor 7–8, 10, 14, 16, 28
    gaps between commissioning parent(s) and surrogate 31, 33, 44
    role in valuation of eggs 32–33
Colen, Shellee 3
colorism 32, 33–36

Egypt
    access to IVF services 38–39
    attitudes to gestational surrogacy 39
    colorism and racism 35–36
    comparable to U.S. regarding disparities in access to ART 38, 50
    financing IVF treatment 37–38
    Islamic religious law and ART 38, 39
embryo disposal 39
**embryo transfer:** the transfer of an embryo from a glass receptacle or from a woman's body to another woman's body with the goal of implantation in the woman's womb 15
"estranged labor" 15–16
ethical issues 2–3, 16
    regarding rights to surrogacy 48–49

**F**
feminists
    Black 8, 14–15
    divided opinion over Baby M case 6–7
    ideological divisions over commercial surrogacy 7, 10
**forced surrogacy:** a system of involuntary and unpaid reproduction that existed in the United States in which enslaved women were denied reproductive liberty and forced to be inseminated (typically involving rape and other forms of sexual violence) by men to whom they were not legally married and to whom their children were commodities. Their bodies were treated as baby factories used to produce commodities that could be sold. They were forced to bear children of whom they would not be the legally recognized parent. This system restricted the reproductive liberty of millions of women of African and multiracial ancestry. 14, 15

**G**
gay men 5
    access to ART 26–27, 45–46, 49
    advertisements targeting 23
    single men advertising for a surrogate 23–24
genetic ties 7, 11, 25–26
Germany 15
gestational carrier
    *see* **gestational surrogate**
**gestational surrogacy/surrogate:** this is the most common form of commercial surrogacy today. The gestational surrogate is the birth mother of a child who is born as

a result of a commercial labor contract. A surrogate who gestates a fetus to whom she has no genetic tie. She agrees to be impregnated and carries the pregnancy to term for an individual or couple who are the "intended" parents by contract. She is a paid laborer working on a nine-month commercial contract 1, 11

## H

## I

**in vitro fertilization (IVF):** literally means "in glass." This refers to a biological process that would ordinarily take place within the body, but instead occurs outside of the body or in a glass Petri dish or other laboratory receptacle. Embryos can be produced by IVF using sperm and/or eggs from third parties (donors, sellers) and then transferred to the body of a surrogate or intended parent. 2, 5, 11

**intended mother (or father):** this is the individual or couple who "contracts" or commissions the birth of the child using ART and signs a preconception labor contract with a surrogate (and/or agency) indicating that they will assume legal and parental responsibility for the child upon birth. This individual is recognized as the legal and social parent of the child regardless of their genetic relationship. In Israel and some U.S. states their name, rather than that of the birth mother appears on the legal birth certificate. 11

Markens, Susan 16, 49
maternal connections 46
maternal mortality rate, India 17
military wives 1–2
Morgan, Derek 30
*Mother Jones* 17
motherhood
    debate on meaning of 49
    deconstructed in surrogacy 10–11, 44
    economic benefits of 16
    Israeli cult of 47

## N
Nahman, Michal 35
*New York Times Magazine* 9–10
*Newsweek* 1–2

## O
Oliver, Kelly 6, 15–16
"Outsourced Wombs" 1
**outsourcing:** to farm out (work), for example to an outside provider or manufacturer, to cut costs 1

## P
Pande, Amrita 45–47, 48
physical characteristics, desirable 32, 33–36
poverty
    and lack of reproductive liberty 16, 37, 41, 50
    a motive to be a surrogate mother 3–4, 9, 16, 46, 48
procreation, right to 50
**procreative liberty:** a primary liberty. It is the right to be free from state intervention in procreative decisions, whether the decision is to have children or to avoid having them (Robertson 1994). In the case of Israel, this is a positive right—that is, the right to have the state or particular persons provide the means or resources necessary to have or avoid having children. 50
    *see also* **reproductive liberty**
**procreative substances:** genetic material that includes sperm and ova (eggs) that is necessary to reproduce a human being 38
**pundekaut:** Hebrew term which means innkeeper. Term used in Israeli courts to define the practice of gestational surrogacy. According to Elly Teman's (2010) analysis this term privileges genetics over gestation and thus minimizes the surro-

gate's influence on the child's development and reduces her role to that of a "host" or vessel. 28

# R

**reproductive liberty:** Dorothy Roberts discusses this in reference to U.S. Black women who have historically been denied the right to determine when and how many children to produce. For most of U.S. history, as slaves, they did not have any rights to their children, who were the property of White male slave owners. 8, 50

**reproductive tourism/surrogacy tourism:** a form of medical tourism. Individuals or couples travel to another state (within the U.S.), region, or nation in order to purchase procreative substances (egg, sperm, embryos) and/or fertility services that include ovum donation, sperm donation, surrogacy arrangements. Individuals travel in order to avoid the legal or regulatory regimes in their nation or to purchase ART services for a cheaper price. For example an individual who lives in Italy, Germany, or Japan where this is banned may travel to the United States,

India, or another European country where these services are legal. 17–18, 26–27, 31, 45

right to privacy 41, 49

Roberts, Dorothy 8, 25–26, 50

*Roe v. Wade* (1973) 4

Roman Catholicism 39

Rosenblatt, Roger 2

Rotabi, Karen Smith 9

## S

same sex couples and access to ART 5, 23, 25, 26, 49

Sanders, Cheryl J. 15

**second shift:** a term that refers to the "double day" that employed working mothers and wives do at home. Arlie Hochschild (2003) found that dual-income married couples with children do not equally divide the domestic labor, which includes cooking, cleaning, child care, shopping, and home maintenance. Women do a disproportionate share of work even when employed full-time outside of the home. 19

**sexualized care work:** refers to a form of labor that involves body parts that are stigmatized and that parallels some aspects of sex work. Amrita Pande introduces this concept to account for the labor of Indian women who work as gestational surrogates. 46

skin color 32, 33–36

slavery

commodification of children 8, 16

and denial of reproductive liberty for women 8, 13–14, 50

and historical commodification of reproduction 14–15

Spar, Deborah 7, 8, 13

sperm donors 18

and consumer choice 33–35

Stern, Elizabeth 5, 6

Stern, William 5, 6

stigma of surrogacy 46–47

**stratified reproduction:** the differential experiences, rewards, and values accorded to reproductive labor based on racial, class, gender, and other inequalities. Racial, ethnic, class, and gender inequalities, and migration status all affect access to material and social resources and this structures who is allowed to reproduce and nurture and the conditions under which they are able to accomplish this. An example would be poor women who migrate to the United States or Europe, leaving their children behind to be fostered while they care for the children of the upper middle classes in another country (see Ginsburg and Rapp 1995). 3, 16, 37

**structural racism:** also referred to as institutional racism. A system of social institutions or social structures including schools, banks, courts, police, and hospitals. Individuals in these institutions can engage in practices that produce cumulative and durable inequalities that are race- or caste-based. These practices reinforce racial and ethnic inequalities that have material consequences for the entire lives of the objects of structural racism. These practices have long-term effects and result in lifetime disadvantage by restricting their educational and employment options. 50

**surrogate:** a substitute, a person standing for another person or thing. A woman who bears a baby for another, especially a childless couple, after IVF or implantation of an embryo. Surrogacy is the practice whereby one woman carries a child for another with the intention that the child will be relinquished after birth to the "intended" parents for a fee. 1

**Surrogate Motherhood Agreements Law:** this law was passed in 1996 in Israel, making it the first and only nation in the world to implement a regulatory regime in which each and every surrogacy contract must be approved by the state. All IVF treatments up to the birth of two children are state-funded. The Surrogate Agreement Law does not give any legal status to the birth mother upon the child's birth. The Law allows only for gestational surrogacy agreements between Israeli citizens who are religiously and ethnically matched. The sperm must be from the "intended" father. 42–43

**surrogate orphan:** a child born who has no legal parents and thus no citizenship. This can occur if the commissioning parents divorce, die, or separate during the pregnancy and there is a disagreement between local authorities and the agency, and no birth certificate can be issued due to confusion about the child's legal parentage. There have been several cases of this in India and Europe, which has called attention to the lack of adequate judicial procedures to handle these cases. 45

**symbolic capital:** coined by Pierre Bourdieu, a 20th century French sociologist who studied social stratification and the reproduction of social inequalities. Symbolic capital is a resource that is associated with prestige or honor. Critical race scholars have argued that in a society such as the United States with a history of race-based slavery and which has been dominated politically and economically by European Americans, whiteness or lighter skin is a form of symbolic capital because it is associated with the racially dominant group and thus with superiority and power. 33–34

**traditional surrogate:** the birth mother is both the "gestational" surrogate and the biological mother. In contrast to those that are just "gestational" surrogates she has a genetic tie to the child she is carrying because she has contributed the ovum. Like a gestational surrogate she is selling her reproductive labor, that is renting her womb out for a fee. In traditional case law she is the legally recognized mother until she relinquishes the child for adoption. 7, 11, 12

**wage exiles:** individuals or couples who must migrate to other countries to secure higher wages and live in exile for long periods of time, maybe several years, in order to secure enough money to pay for assisted reproductive technologies such as IVF, embryo transfers, or other procedures that are expensive. 38